They Call Me "Doctor Death"

They Call Me "Doctor Death"

*How Our Medical System
Robs the Terminally Ill
of Comfort, Time, and Dignity*

Dr. Ken Pettit

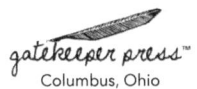

Columbus, Ohio

They Call Me "Doctor Death":
How Our Medical System Robs the Terminally Ill of Comfort,
Time, and Dignity

Published by Gatekeeper Press
2167 Stringtown Rd, Suite 109
Columbus, OH 43123-2989
www.GatekeeperPress.com

Copyright © 2021 by Ken Petitt

All rights reserved. Neither this book, nor any parts within it may be sold or reproduced in any form or by any electronic or mechanical means, including information storage and retrieval systems without permission in writing from the author. The only exception is by a reviewer, who may quote short excerpts in a review.

LCCN: 2021933020

ISBN (hardcover): 9781662908934
ISBN (paperback): 9781662906008
ISBN (eBook): 9781662916496

Dedication

To my fiancé Megan, my parents, brothers and
sisters, children and grandchildren,
my grandson Parker, and my dear friend Steve.

To my wonderful team and many other staff
members I've worked with over the years.

We are all in this together.

And to the patients and families
I have cared for over the years.

How honored I am for being a part of your lives
at a very special time.

Contents

Introduction
They Call Me "Doctor Death" 1

Chapter One
You Don't Have to Do This.. 9

Chapter Two
A Day in the Life 21

Chapter Three
You're Getting Better (But Still Dying) 37

Chapter Four
Death Doesn't Cure Dysfunction: Why Advance
Planning is Crucial 57

Chapter Five
Technology Makes it Hard to Die 69

Chapter Six
The Death Talk... 77

Chapter Seven
The Money Game (or You're Not Dying Fast Enough) 93

Chapter Eight
How to Make Doctors Work for You 105

Chapter Nine
Recommendations for Change 123

Epilogue 143

Acknowledgments 147

Resources for Readers 149

About the Author 151

Index 153

INTRODUCTION

They Call Me "Doctor Death"

I was eating lunch in the doctors' lounge one day when in walked a physician I'll call Dr. X. He placed his hand on my shoulder and, with a half-smile on his face, turned to the other doctors in the room.

"How many of you want to see Dr. Pettit visiting *your* patient?" he called out. "You all know what he does here—he's the *last* person you want to put on your case! Who in their right mind wants a visit from Doctor Death?"

Laughter rose around me, spilling through the room. I tried to join in, hiding my discomfort the way you do when Uncle Joe says something crazy at Thanksgiving dinner. The labels pinned on me varied—*Grim Reaper, Angel of Death, Prince of Darkness*—but the uneasiness I felt on hearing them never changed.

Dr. X is just being facetious, I told myself as the laughter petered out and the doctors went back to their hurried lunches. After all, he was one of my biggest advocates. He worked in the ICU and called me in all the time to handle the most difficult cases.

"Ken, this patient is not in a good place," he would tell me. "I'll do everything I can do to save him because that's what his family wants me to do, but we both know he's going to die pretty soon. I need you to establish some sort of plan. I can put in another tube, I can do another test, I can throw another drug at him, but we both know it's futile. Please, Ken—go talk to him as soon as you can."

Dr. X does a good job handling his side of it, and I do a good job handling my side. Other doctors can talk about the next test or the next procedure, about a prognosis and possible progress. Other doctors can say, "I'm doing the full-court press. I'm doing everything I possibly can to help you pull through." But I'm the "other doctor"—the one who bears the news that medicine can't fix the loved one's broken body, that reality has overtaken hope, that there's nothing more to be done.

I'm not a heart surgeon, an oncologist, or a neurologist. Rather, as a palliative and hospice care physician, I work with patients, both in and outside the hospital, who have advanced incurable diseases and are terminal (defined as having six months or less to live). I have my own hospice company with a staff of nurses, social workers, chaplains, certified nursing assistants, volunteers, and bereavement counselors who visit dying patients and their families. My goal is to prevent and relieve suffering for these patients, whether they choose to continue treatment or make the transition to hospice and "comfort measures," where the focus is not on prolonging life but on helping them die a dignified death with as little physical and emotional suffering as possible.

Every day, I help patients face the choice of whether to continue treatment or to allow death to naturally unfold, so they can have the best possible quality of life up to the end.

It's never an easy conversation to have, and I've had it thousands of times. I don't want to take away their hope, but I don't want to rob patients of precious time by making false promises. Most seriously ill patients think they have to accept every possible treatment and procedure. They get caught up in the momentum of a life-prolonging system that performs every procedure and treats every symptom. I'm there to help them understand that they don't have to go down that road, that they can accept death and use the days they have left to prepare for it.

But far too many doctors don't understand or embrace what I do. I'm called "Doctor Death" or "The Grim Reaper" because I'm the one with the bad news, who carts their patients off to hospice. I'm the fly in the ointment, the shadow on the wall, the person they try to avoid. I make them uncomfortable because I go against the grain of a medical establishment that views death as an enemy to be fought and defeated rather than as an inevitable and natural part of life that should be respected, not feared. My work challenges a medical establishment that routinely promotes aggressive treatments to the very end of life, which, in the majority of cases, only prolongs suffering for both patients and their families, preventing the terminally ill from dying "a good death."

Yes, we've learned to cure a wide range of illnesses, allowing countless people to live longer lives. But our medical powers are neither infinite nor infallible. Each year, thousands of people older than eighty-five die in intensive care units while undergoing futile treatments.

A 2017 Kaiser Family Foundation poll found that seven in ten Americans say they would prefer to die at home, yet according to a study by the *Journal of Palliative Medicine*, about 71% of Americans have little to no understanding of palliative and hospice care. And close to 60% of patients who would benefit from palliative care never receive it (*New England Journal of Medicine*). Those who do are in hospice for too short a time to receive its full benefits. According to the National Hospice and Palliative Care Organization (NHPCO), in 2017, about 40% of hospice patients were in hospice for less than two weeks.

No one wants to die, but some ways of dying are far better than others. You can meet your end hooked up to a machine. You can deny the reality of your mortality, or you can find peace with death in the comfort of hospice care, where the process of death is natural.

I've been pretty good at helping people die a good death during my career, and it doesn't have anything to do with my knowledge of medicine. I like to think that I'm a knowledgeable physician, but what I do best is connect and communicate with dying patients and their families. I'm able to openly talk about a subject few of us want to discuss.

My work is difficult, not because I have difficult conversations about death, but because I'm prevented from having those conversations until it's too late. You can do chemotherapy and radiation and all the treatments you want because everyone wants to live another day. But while you're chasing after that goal, you lose the opportunity to be at peace with whatever life you have left.

The Covid-19 pandemic brought these end-of-life issues into stark and heartbreaking focus. Families couldn't be with their dying loved ones to ease their passing. Doctors did their best to counsel family members via Zoom. And as cases mounted amid a national shortage of personal protective equipment, with doctors and nurses constantly exposed to a highly infectious disease, some health professionals began to question the value and morality of using every last procedure on severely ill and terminal patients.

That's why I wanted to write this book—to help people understand that we have the option to prepare for our deaths in an early and proactive way, rather than accept treatments and procedures that only prolong suffering.

In the following pages, I look closely at my personal and professional experience with death. I examine problems in our current medical system and offer suggestions on how that system can be changed for the better. This is not a theoretical book or one focused solely on medical policy; rather, it's based on my experiences with hundreds of patients and families. Throughout this book, I refer again and again to specific people I've worked with over the years (all names have been changed for reasons of privacy).

Among the major themes I address are the following:

- How watching friends and family die influenced my views on how the dying should be treated.
- How dysfunction, denial, and deception permeate our treatment of the terminally ill.
- How suffering is routinely prolonged because we fear talking realistically about death.
- How hope is oversold, leading dying patients into believing that they're getting better.
- How medical technology often prevents terminal patients from "dying a good death."
- How financial accountability is either misused or absent from our medical system in treating the seriously ill or hospice patients.
- How physicians and caregivers can improve the ways they communicate and interact with patients around end-of-life issues.
- How the average person can be empowered to ask questions and challenge assumptions about their care when nearing the end of life.

- The crucial importance of advance planning—how everyone should have in place advance directives and a designated medical power of attorney (MPOA).

We're all terrified of death, but we're dying from the moment we're conceived. If someone says to me, "Aunt Sue is not dying," my response is gentle but direct.

"Well, every one of us is dying, so let's take that off the table."

If a patient has been in the hospital nine times, the reality is that she probably would have died at least two or three times had we not intervened. We don't give the patient and family the opportunity to get off that crazy train. So, yes, the patient is dying. They're dying of their disease and we keep getting in the way.

The hospital is a terrible place to meet your end. We don't do death well. We start too late to prepare for it and we focus on the wrong things. We want to control something we can't control, and we experience unnecessary and destructive guilt as a result. If someone sends their loved one to hospice, that person can come to believe that they've sentenced their loved one to death. But death is as natural as birth, and a large part of my job is helping families accept that fact. Hospice is not a death sentence but a service that helps people die as comfortably as possible.

The issues I face every day and that I address in this book are nuanced and complicated. Doctors are trained to save lives, to use every means and technology they have to preserve life. The families of the seriously ill and dying often want to see everything possible done to save their loved ones. It's not easy to make decisions when you're in a hospital bed. In the abstract, we can say that we don't want to pursue further treatment, but we may change our minds when death is near. Until you're wearing those shoes, you don't know what you're going to do.

But if we all die someday, we have the power to choose the best way for that to happen. I hope this book helps everyone—patients, families, and medical professionals—break our collective silence about death, so we can develop better ways of talking about, treating, and encountering what we will all someday face.

Dr. Ken Pettit
Jan. 1, 2021

CHAPTER ONE

You Don't Have to Do This

Steve was my best friend. I was nineteen when I met him through our mutual love of motorcycles. About six years older than me, he quickly became the older brother I never had. We rode thousands of miles throughout the West on our Harleys, sometimes 300 miles a day, the wind whipping our hair and the sun burning our faces in those wide-open spaces.

I was in college at the time, taking pre-med classes while working as a hospital orderly, hoping to go to medical school someday. Steve was a police officer, and his work had the same quality that attracted me to medicine—helping people in crisis. I became more and more drawn to law enforcement and eventually became a reserve officer in the same department where Steve worked. When offered a full-time job on the force, I grabbed it.

I loved my new career, whether it was helping victims of a car accident, intervening in domestic violence, or preventing a robbery. There was a thrill to the work, an adrenaline rush I couldn't deny. My best friend and I were working together and motorcycling on weekends, living life to the fullest.

But after two years on the force, my urge to go to medical school kept nagging at me, and Steve knew it.

"This job isn't the real you," he told me one day. "If you stay in police work much longer, you'll never leave. It's a hard job to walk away from—the pay is good, you'll have a family someday, you'll be able to retire in twenty years, and you'll be hooked. Those twenty years will flash right by, and you'll wonder where they went. If you truly want to be a doctor, Ken, you need to get out now before the job consumes you."

An "ah-ha" moment, big time. I left the police department, became a paramedic who drove ambulances and flew in helicopters, and then a registered nurse working in the emergency room. I finished college and was accepted into med school. Throughout this big shift in my life, Steve and I stayed good friends.

Since he was six years older than me, he was getting close to retirement age while I was still studying to be a doctor. Nearing the end of his law enforcement career, he decided that he wanted to become a physician's assistant (P.A.). He was accepted to my medical school just as I finished my academics and was doing rotations. We were living next door to each other, having good times when we weren't busy with our training.

During Steve's second year in the P.A. program, he began to change a bit. One time, he asked me to help him with a very simple thing, getting a garage door unstuck. It caught me off guard. Steve was a very handy guy—he took motorcycles apart and put them back together—but I figured he was just stressed out.

Not long after that, on his way back from a rotation, his truck got a flat tire and he couldn't remember how to change it.

Throughout our more than ten years of friendship, he

never forgot my birthday—a card, a letter, a phone call, a meal. But, for the first time, my birthday came and went without a word from him.

One night, I got a frantic call from his wife. Steve had had a seizure at home and was taken to the hospital. The diagnosis: a huge brain tumor. He was only forty, a very young man.

I was in my fourth year of medical school, he was in the second year of his P.A. program, and we had been scheduled to graduate at the same time. Our plan was to open a little medical practice together and do the work that we loved best for the rest of our careers. Now, in a very short time, those best-laid plans slipped upside down.

Steven underwent brain surgery and radiation. There wasn't a lot of chemotherapy available at the time for the type of cancer he had. The doctors were chasing after a cure that didn't exist.

When I graduated from medical school, he was pretty debilitated, able to walk only with a cane (he was too proud to use the walker he really needed), yet he had his wife drive him to my graduation ceremony, the one we were supposed to attend together.

When I was ready to walk across the stage, I glanced up at the stands but couldn't find him. I knew he was there, watching me graduate, knowing all the while that his name wouldn't be called.

As I started my internship and residency, which were pretty grueling, Steve's disease continued to progress. He could no longer walk and became bed-ridden. He was confused much of the time and couldn't remember basic things.

During my evenings off, I spent the night at his house to give his wife some relief, an hour to go grocery shopping or to decompress. I'd help her turn him or get him into the shower—Steve was a big guy, 6' 4" and 220 pounds. I helped him clean himself, dried and dressed him, and got him back into bed.

You can get very restless when you're dying. Steve would ask me to help him sit up, and a moment later, he wanted to lie flat. "Turn me," he'd ask. A moment later: "Don't turn me." I could never get him comfortable. We'd circle around and around his conflicting wishes, trapped in a tormenting, never-ending loop.

By now, I was officially a doctor but had received zero training in how to deal with death. I was learning how to diagnose people and how to fix and cure them, but I didn't have a clue about how to prepare my best friend and his wife for what was coming next.

There was so much I wished I had known as Steve was dying. I didn't know what to say to them. I didn't know how to act around them. I didn't know how to help a dying person face his end. I was plagued with survivor's guilt. Steve and I had the best-laid plans. We'd open our medical practice and be the dynamic duo we'd always been. I still had my whole life ahead of me, and Steve had a few weeks at best.

All the shopworn clichés about death passed through my head:

"You need to push on with your life."

"It's okay not to feel guilty."

"You'll learn to live with the loss, and someday you'll benefit from it."

Empty clichés that meant not a particle of sense. I was emotionally bereft. As a doctor, I had been trained to save the world, but I was helpless to save Steve.

He eventually declined to the point where he was unresponsive in a hospital bed.

Unbelievably, I didn't know what hospice was. I knew it was a place you were referred to when you were getting ready to die, but that was about it. Never had I taken a course about or been trained in end-of-life issues. I knew nothing about the philosophies of hospice, the premises on which it operated, or the services it provided.

The goal of hospice is to make sure that you have some sort of peace and acceptance in facing death, whether you're the patient or the family. Steve didn't receive that support. He wasn't visited by a social worker or chaplain. I didn't know either was available. A nurse came by to give him various medications, but preparing someone to die takes much more than that.

Studies show it takes several months. Steve had about two weeks. He was in terminal condition with brain cancer. He had earned a black belt in karate. We rode Harleys together for thousands of miles. In his prime, he was 220 pounds. Now he weighed maybe 100 pounds at best and could no longer speak. I had my whole life ahead of me while he had lost everything.

He wasn't eating. He wasn't drinking. His urine output wasn't there. His wife discussed putting in an IV.

"He'll die if he becomes dehydrated," she told me. "We've got to give him something."

She convinced me to take that step. He was unresponsive, couldn't eat, and had lost over a hundred pounds. It was my job to keep him alive. We made arrangements and Steve underwent a procedure to give him long-term IV access.

One night Steve's IV stopped and it freaked me out. The finality of his death was upon us.

I put a stethoscope to his chest and heard a horrible heart murmur. Yet, I was still medically intellectualizing my best friend's impending death, deceiving myself into thinking I was saving him when there was no chance of that. He wasn't dying from kidney failure due to dehydration; he was dying from brain cancer. And yet, I was injecting him full of saline, syringe by syringe, two teaspoons at a time through his failing IV, until he got a liter of fluid into his system. Because that's what I knew, what I had been trained to do—to try everything to the bitter end.

His wife was also in denial, completely focused on IV fluids to keep her husband from dying. No one talked to her about the range of complex feelings I now discuss with patients as a hospice physician. No one talked to her about allowing the natural process of dying to occur.

Instead of stopping treatment, dealing with his wife's emotions, and making Steve as comfortable as possible in his last days, I fell into a desperate tunnel vision. We couldn't have him die from kidney failure. I had to give his wife every last bit of hope. I had to make sure he got his IV fluids.

Soon, his IV got totally plugged up and we couldn't use it anymore. Steve went into renal failure, and within a week, he passed away. My actions hadn't prolonged his life for more than a couple of days at best.

Today, instead of aggressively treating a terminal case up to the end, I would have made Steve and his wife as comfortable as possible. I would have helped them accept his passage. I would have given them time to process his death rather than deny it. This would have allowed them to go through what Herb Knoll, author of *The Widower's Journey*, calls "anticipatory grief" or "pre-grief," a period that gives loved ones the time to gradually adjust to the reality of a coming death.

But I did none of those things because I didn't know about

them. This was a hard lesson to learn, and it wasn't just Steve who taught it to me.

My father came from a family with a long history of lung disease. To make matters worse, he grew up in an era where everyone smoked—in cars, in airplanes, in front of children. And dad was in the military, where one of the only things to do was smoke.

I was still in medical school when my father ended up on oxygen because of COPD (chronic obstructive pulmonary disease). He was only in his early or mid-fifties, and yet the outlook for his life expectancy wasn't good.

While he was undergoing treatment, there were a lot of advances in treating lung disease, including lung transplants. Because of his close relationship with my mom, he wanted to give her every hope and decided to take that very aggressive route.

Dad went through living hell to get on the transplant list. While battling his COPD, he ended up getting prostate cancer. You have to be free of cancer for five years or more before you can get a transplant. He also had a heart attack, so he had to be deemed recovered and healthy enough for such a major operation. If someone can't walk two feet to go to the bathroom, you can't put that person on a table, crack open his chest, and replace his lungs. You've got to have a lot left in the tank to recover. Dad was hospitalized for months, in and out of the ICU, until he finally met the criteria to get on the transplant list.

We lived in Phoenix, and he had to go to Tucson for the operation. He lived in an apartment near the hospital for three months so he could make his frequent medical appointments.

He seemed to do fairly well for a period of time and was

able to move back to Phoenix, but then he became extremely sick from the medication that prevented his body from rejecting the transplant. He was flown by helicopter back to the Tucson medical center and was in the ICU, on and off a ventilator numerous times. He returned to Phoenix, had another setback, and was again flown by helicopter down to Tucson's ICU unit.

After an especially rough day, the two of us began to talk about the end of his life. I said to him, "You know, dad, you don't have to keep going through this."

I didn't say it because I was a hospice doctor. I said it because I couldn't stand to see him suffer anymore. He was such a good guy, such a personable man. Everyone loved my dad. How much more could he take? How much more did he want to take? It was a conversation I wish I had been able to have with Steve fifteen years before.

Dad looked at me and said, "I'm not going to let your mom down. I'm going to keep fighting." After a pause, he went on. "But when the time comes and I'm stuck on that machine, and there's no chance that I'm going to recover, I don't want you to leave me on it for more than a minute longer than I need to be. Because if you do, I'm going to come back and haunt you until the day you die. And when I see you again in the next world, I'm going to kick your ass. So remember what I said, Ken—do not leave me on the machine if you know I'm not going to make it."

At that time, someone with a lung transplant has a 50% chance of living for five years if they get past the first year. The day before dad's big milestone, his first anniversary, he had an appointment at the Phoenix clinic.

I told my mom, "Great. Just keep me posted on how everything goes."

That night, at 3 a.m., I got a call from her. "Your dad just went into cardiac arrest. I did CPR on him, called 911, and he's on the way to the hospital."

I was dumbfounded.

"What the hell happened? Didn't he have an appointment at the clinic just a few hours ago?"

"No, they canceled it."

I blew a cork. "What do you mean they canceled it?"

"They called and said they were really busy and running behind, and they didn't want him to wait in a chair for hours. Your dad had a fever and was feeling pretty bad, but he felt there were people worse off who needed to see a doctor more than he did."

I couldn't believe it. "He's a lung transplant patient with a fever and they didn't insist he come in??"

Later, when I talked with his doctor, he said it was a miscommunication. At any rate, had dad had the cardiac arrest at the clinic, his prognosis wouldn't have been better. He had a temperature of 103, so I knew he was septic at that point. He was in the ICU and back on a ventilator.

There's a procedure called a "hypothermia protocol" that can be used to treat someone in dad's condition. You put the patient under a cooling blanket to drop their core temperature. When you warm them back up, you'll sometimes see improved neurological function. Some people (not many) have recovered enough to go home. My mom wanted to try it, to give dad every last chance. She needed the peace of mind that she had tried absolutely everything, and for her sake, I went along with it.

When they warmed him back up and did their neurological testing, dad had minimal brain function. He was completely unresponsive and helpless. Although he could no longer speak to me, I had the feeling he was looking for a way out, and

I had to give it to him. I remembered what he had told me: "Do not leave me on the machine if you know I'm not going to make it."

One of the intensive care doctors walked in and said to me, "Ken, you know where this is at and where it's going. Do you really want to keep doing this?"

I called a meeting with my mom and one of my three siblings and communicated with dad's brothers. I told them what dad had said to me. "And now we're here. He's not going to get better. He's not who he was anymore, and we need to shut this down."

My mom and my brother agreed. My other brother couldn't be there. When he married his wife at eighteen, she was already on dialysis; she died at thirty-seven after being in the ICU more times than my brother could remember.

"Ken, I can't go through this again," he told me. "I can't watch dad die. I went through it so many times before."

He hadn't found peace because his wife had never been in hospice. She was in the ICU right up to her death. She went through heart surgery just weeks before she passed. Neither she nor my brother had the time to fully prepare for her passing.

My sister couldn't be there either because she wanted to remember my father as he was. People find closure in their own unique ways.

After talking with my family, mom and I and my brother went into dad's room and shut the machine off. I thought it was ironic that his lungs were functioning with textbook perfection, keeping his body alive, and now I had turned off the ventilator. His lungs—his lifelong nemesis—were doing great, and still we couldn't save him.

Three or four minutes passed, and I heard the alarm go off at the nurse's station. A couple of minutes later, the doctor came in and pronounced him dead. I had my grief, but I also had my peace.

To this day, I feel my dad picked his time. Not consciously, not in a way we can understand, but he chose his day. He died two weeks before my parents were to celebrate their fiftieth anniversary. I believe he knew it was coming; he had purchased a gift for my mom and put it away for her, which we found after he passed.

My father had been through hell and back. He had suffered enough, and perhaps he felt we had suffered enough with him. I will always think he picked his moment.

As with Steve, much of my father's suffering was needless and prolonged. He told me multiple times when we were alone: "I'm tired. I'm not sure how much more I can do this. But your mom is telling me I've got to keep fighting, that I can beat this." And so his fight became a performance for her.

I carry the experiences of Steve and my dad with me as I help families deal with death. I understand what they're going through because I've walked in their shoes. I never mention Steve or my dad when I speak to them. I don't say that I had a friend who was pumped full of fluids during the last two weeks of his life, only prolonging his agony. Or that my dad went through living hell to get a lung transplant. I don't bring up my personal history because the focus is on the family, and we all have to find our private ways to deal with mortality. But what happened to Steve and my father is always with me in my work.

Today, when I talk to a patient who is near the end of life, I close the door when no one is around and say, "Do you want to keep going?" I say it straight and they know exactly what I'm talking about.

And sometimes they'll tell me, "I can't do it. I can't keep going."

"You don't have to do it."

These are the words that set them free, and that freedom enables us to open a dialog together. I'm able to understand who they are, what they want, and what I need to do to advocate for them, to be their voice. I'm able to start working to bring everyone in the family together, so their loved one can die with dignity and the least possible pain.

CHAPTER TWO

A Day in the Life

Recently, in the course of a single day, I met with four patients whose cases epitomized the dysfunction, denial, and deception that characterize our treatment of the terminally ill.

The first was Robert, a sixty-four-year-old gentleman with a history of Lupus, kidney failure, and heart problems. He came into the hospital because he was septic due to an infection from his pacemaker. They had to remove it, he started having problems with bleeding, and his platelet count went down. A kidney transplant he had the year before had failed, so he was back on dialysis.

When admitted to the ICU, Robert's heart would stop beating for ten or fifteen seconds before it resumed a normal rhythm. Too sick to have a pacemaker reinstalled permanently, Robert's doctors decided to install a temporary one in his groin. While doing so, his other systems started to fail. Robert's infection was under control, but he was still on dialysis and his blood count started to go down. After two weeks in the ICU, he couldn't do much more than lie flat; now and then, he could sit up to about 30 degrees. He was incontinent and soiled himself in bed.

His doctors' goal had been to treat him with antibiotics

so they could put in a permanent pacemaker and send him to rehab. That never became an option because of Robert's multitude of problems. The physicians understood that he would die whether or not he received a permanent pacemaker, so I got the call to see him.

We had had a good talk the week before. He was tired of years of aggressive treatment, and we discussed his wishes should he end up on a ventilator: "If there's nothing they can do, why am I laying here in bed losing precious time? I want to go home and spend time with my family and play with my grandkids."

Robert and I agreed on this goal. Understanding that nothing more could be done, we changed his resuscitation status so he wouldn't end up on a machine or be needlessly subjected to CPR. Robert's wife, Jane, wasn't present when I had the initial conversation with him. The next day, she dropped by to visit while I went to see another patient.

When I returned about an hour later, Robert and Jane were eating in his room. When I greeted them, Jane said curtly, "I know why *you're* here."

Feeling that I was interrupting, I told them I could come back after they finished their meal.

"That's okay," Jane said, her words tinged with anger. "I just lost my appetite." She set down her tray. "The doctors told me they had plans to treat him. Now all of a sudden, you walk in here and the plans have changed. That's just not acceptable to me!"

As Robert listened, I did my best to respond.

"Please understand that we don't have any new options to explore. We've tried everything. The doctors have told you there's nothing more we can do. We don't want Robert's life to end here in the hospital. We can keep him alive, plugged into all these machines, lying flat in that bed, but that's going to be the extent of his life from here on out. Your husband has made his wishes clear. He wants to go home and spend time with you and your family, and I don't think we should change that plan to accommodate expectations that are unrealistic."

Jane was unmoved.

"You're telling me that, even if they do more things, he's still going to die? Really? Then we're going to find a different doctor and a different hospital! There's got to be *some* doctor out there who can treat him!"

"Jane, are you saying that your husband needs to stay plugged into a machine until he dies, something he doesn't want? There's probably someone out there who *will* do that, but based on everything we've discussed, it's not going to happen at this facility."

Jane stood up. "Well, we'll see about that. I'm calling one of my kids!"

As Robert and I listened, she screamed into the phone at her stepdaughter.

"They just came in and told us there's nothing more they can do, that he just needs to go home and die! Can you believe it? These doctors are giving up on him—they're going to discharge him right into the streets. But they're not getting away with that—we need to call a lawyer and find a new doctor!"

On speakerphone, Robert and I overheard the stepdaughter's equally enraged response.

"I want him moved to a different hospital so they can do this procedure! If not, tell Dr. Pettit I'm going to sue him, the other doctors, and the hospital too!"

I couldn't bear that Robert was listening to all this—a patient with Lupus, a failed kidney transplant, who had sepsis and was on dialysis. His wife and daughter were perfectly okay moving him to another hospital, where new doctors would prolong his life for a few days at best, subjecting him to all kinds of painful procedures.

"If Robert dies, he dies," the stepdaughter screamed into the phone, "but then at least I'm okay with it! At least we've done everything and not given up on him!"

Three days before, when I met Jane for the first time, she had told me that she was under a lot of stress, trying to fit her visits to the ICU in between chemotherapy treatments for her Stage 4 terminal colon cancer.

When she got off the phone, I said, "Jane, please listen to me. If somebody was telling you how to manage your chemotherapy, how would you react to that?"

"That's not fair," she replied.

I didn't let her off the hook. "So you're telling me you wouldn't let your stepdaughter dictate your chemo treatment, but you're telling me it's acceptable for you to control your husband?"

"But there are still things they can do to him!"

We were splitting hairs. She was blowing the wind any way she wanted it to blow. And so I left, hoping I could visit Robert alone the next day to tell him he had the right and the ability to die in the way he wanted.

I drove to another hospital to visit Gene, eighty-one, who suffered from Parkinson's and dementia and had been on a ventilator at home for eight years. He had had multiple ICU admissions over those eight years. This time, he had been in the ICU for two weeks. Up to this point, all his doctors had been on board: *tune him up, get him out, tune him up again, get him out again.* Now, when things seemed out of hand, they no longer wanted to put Gene through all this torment. I was called in to visit him for the first time. How quickly could I get him out of there and into hospice?

I could have started that process three or four months before. Maybe we would have prevented Gene from going through four more hospitalizations. Maybe we could have set the stage for a compassionate end-of-life plan. But now, I had only a few days to accomplish these emotionally fraught and psychologically complicated tasks.

Gene's first wife had died some years before. They had one son, Carl, and Gene had since been remarried to Vivian. When Gene started to decline, he and Vivian realized his care was going to cost a lot of money. He had created a lot of wealth but didn't want to spend it, and certainly not on his healthcare.

Gene's son Carl told me that his father and stepmother got divorced solely to protect those assets. Gene transferred all his money and property to Vivian and gave her power of attorney to manage them. On paper, Gene was now penniless and unable to pay for his healthcare. He qualified for state health insurance as well as for the services of a full-time caregiver.

In Arizona, if someone is indigent, the state will pay for a full-time caregiver, and that person can be a family member. The reasoning is that a relative will have the motivation and resources to provide quality care. Vivian applied and was approved. She would be paid $15 an hour for a forty-hour week to care for her husband, while at the same time, owning all of his assets.

Carl told me that Gene had been subjected to treatment after treatment during the previous eight years and had been resuscitated numerous times whenever his heart stopped. He said Vivian continued to put his father through all this trauma simply to collect a paycheck.

"If she could, my stepmother would keep him plugged into a ventilator for the next ten years," Carl said, "just to game the system."

Whenever a family member questioned her, he said her response was the same: "I've got power of attorney." That was the hospital's view as well: Vivian was legally the boss.

The day before I visited, Gene's doctors had concluded that nothing more could be done and that he should be moved to a place where he could pass. Vivian thought he should die in the hospital; Carl disagreed because of his father's religious beliefs, telling me, "His spirit is going to be released at the time of death, and I don't want his spirit in this hospital. I want him at home. That's where he's always told me he wanted to die. And so it's my duty to respect my father's wishes."

Carl was trying to be the responsible son, but his father's wishes weren't going to happen because Vivian had power of attorney. Gene was slated to die in the hospital.

I found out that Vivian's power of attorney document had been scanned into the hospital's database as part of Gene's living will. Making sure to cover all the bases, I did a little digging and found it. It gave Vivian financial power to manage Gene's stocks, bonds, real estate, and bank account, but in bold letters at the top were the words: "THIS DOCUMENT DOES NOT PERTAIN TO MEDICAL POWER OF ATTORNEY (MPOA)."

For eight years, Vivian had been falsely claiming she had the legal right to make medical decisions for Gene. Apparently, no one had bothered to read the document. Based on Arizona state law, it was Gene's son Carl who had always held MPOA.

When I handed Carl his father's living will, years of anger and frustration blew up in my face.

"Are you serious? Are you shitting me? She's been putting my dad through hell for the last eight years just for a paycheck—and she doesn't have MPOA?! The hospital said they accepted the document! And now you're telling me this?! Doesn't the hospital have any liability for taking Vivian's word and not checking the documents she supplied?"

Carl was inches away, screaming at me. Well, not quite at me, but at everything his father has gone through for no reason. It wasn't easy to endure his rage, but I understood it. All along, he could have been guiding his father toward more compassionate care and a dignified end (ironically, Carl was a family law attorney).

When Carl finally regained control, he said curtly, "I want my dad to die in his own bed, in his own house. Period. End of sentence. No more discussion."

Sounded logical and legal, but guess what? It was Vivian who owned Gene's house, not the son. If Gene was sent home in an ambulance hooked up to a ventilator, accompanied by a registered nurse and a critical care team—sent home with all the resources he needed to survive a fifteen-minute trip so he could die at home—it was Vivian who had the power to stop him at the front door.

Unless Vivian changed her stance, his dad would die in an ambulance parked at the front curb.

During the rest of the day, my phone blew up with text messages as Vivian and Carl waged their war of wills. *Get Gene out of the hospital now! Don't you dare take Gene out of the hospital—or else. Sign this form for me. If you don't do what I say, I'll sue! When is he leaving the hospital? When are you turning off the machine? How quickly can you get him out? What time is the ambulance going to be here? If you dare take him home, you'll hear from my lawyer!*

The next morning, Carl insisted that Gene be transported home, but he refused to pay for the ambulance.

"Let Vivian pay for it. She got everything from my dad—she can afford it!"

Of course, Vivian refused. Carl, on "principle," wouldn't budge. Gene died in the hospital.

As of this writing, Carl is planning to sue Vivian for every dollar she has, to pay back the State of Arizona for all the caregiver dollars she received "caring" for his father. Based on Vivian's forty-hour week at $15 an hour over eight years, that figure came to $249,600.

On the same day that Carl found out about Vivian's phony MPOA, I got a call from a physician at one of the other hospitals where I work. They had a patient who'd been in the hospital for two weeks. Ralph had Parkinson's disease, was wheelchair-bound, and had multiple hospitalizations for aspiration (breathing food and saliva into his airways). He had declined to the point where he couldn't eat or drink anything, so his doctors wanted to put in a feeding tube. In the medical profession, everyone wants to put in a feeding tube, even though it doesn't prevent half the stuff doctors are trying to prevent. The only thing it does in the setting of end-of-life care is stop someone from taking any food by mouth for the rest of his or her life.

Ralph's attending physician couldn't get through to the family, so she called me and said, "Can you talk to his daughter?" I found Anne to be highly educated, extremely articulate, and terribly misinformed.

"We've decided that we're going to go with the feeding tube," she said, "because I don't want him to choke to death on his own vomit."

"What do you mean?"

"Well, I was told that he's already starting to aspirate a little bit, and if he doesn't get the feeding tube, he's going to die of dehydration, choke to death, or starve to death. So we want the feeding tube."

I said, "You need to understand that the feeding tube does not guarantee that he's not going to continue to aspirate. What it does guarantee is that your father, who's awake and alert right now, is never going to take anything by mouth again."

"Somebody told us he could get therapy to teach him how to swallow."

"The problem is that your father's disease has progressed to the point where we can put him through a lot of things to try to accomplish very little. Even with therapy, he'll never get the green light to start eating and drinking again because of his terrible aspiration problems."

Anne held her ground, repeating her three mantras: "I don't want him to starve to death, choke to death, or die from dehydration."

Where had they come from? Maybe she talked to a nurse or a resident. Maybe she Googled "aspiration." Wherever she had found her information, it was now gospel. If you have a loved one in the hospital and a medical professional tells you he's going to choke or starve to death without a feeding tube, you're going to want one.

But a feeding tube doesn't prevent those risks from happening. Instead, too often, it provides the illusion that death can be defeated, an illusion that Anne had entirely bought into.

I've had family members say to me, "All mom loved to do was eat. If we take that away from her, she might as well be dead. That's what she would tell us if she could speak. Go ahead and put it in. It's only temporary, and with physical therapy, she might be able to eat again."

The medicine does not support that that's ever going to happen, so people are being misled. If you can't guarantee that food won't go into your lungs, you shouldn't be eating by mouth. But a feeding tube carries its own risks. As I explain to people, you can't squirt mashed potatoes and gravy in there. It's not that easy. You have to feed him or her a formula based on what the body's going to tolerate and the person's nutritional needs.

What if a bed-bound person gets enough nutrition with a feeding tube, but suffers from horrific diarrhea or constipation? What if the family is told the procedure is temporary when it's likely to be permanent?

Dying patients who are treated appropriately do not experience hunger or dehydration. Palliative care physicians can educate family and medical staff about these truths, but I hadn't been brought in soon enough. Anne was basing monumental end-of-life decisions on her illusions, not reality.

Unable to resolve the impasse with Anne, I left the hospital. In the parking lot, I got a call from Ted, the husband of my patient Marie.

"I'm very worried, Dr. Pettit. Marie is extremely confused, not making any sense." I told him I was on my way.

She'd been in the hospital for forty-five days, having been admitted for a broken leg after a fall. Sent to a rehab facility, she developed an infection and had to return to the hospital, where she went into congestive heart failure and ended up going through dialysis for a few weeks. Marie's kidneys improved and they returned her to rehab. Less than twenty-four hours later, she developed breathing problems and ended up back in the hospital's ICU with renal failure. Marie was dying.

When I arrived at the hospital, it was obvious she had had enough. She was agitated and unable to make decisions for herself. As Ted and I stood at her bedside, he said to me,

"Don't put her on a breathing machine. Don't intubate her, don't do CPR, don't put her back on dialysis. She's tired of all this." The attending doctor agreed that Marie wouldn't be put on a ventilator. I had a bed readied for her in a new facility, so she could have hospice during her final days.

As we were discussing these details, Marie's son Eddie (the stepson of Ted, her second husband) walked into the room. Only later did I learn that this was his first visit to his mother during her six-week hospitalization, while Ted was at Marie's bedside daily from six a.m. until the evening.

"You need to do everything you can to save her," Eddie told me.

"Everything has been done," I said. "She's in kidney failure again, along with congestive heart failure and respiratory failure."

"You're killing my mom," Eddie fired back, "because there's still something you can do for her and you're not doing it!"

A huge argument broke out between Eddie and Ted, with me caught in the middle, while Marie lay unresponsive in bed.

"You're withholding care, you're giving up, you're being selfish!" Eddie screamed at Ted. "She's just a burden to you!"

He stormed out of the hospital and filed a complaint with Adult Protective Services, stating that Ted was depriving his mother of appropriate healthcare. When this didn't work, he filed an emergency injunction with the court, disputing Ted's medical power of attorney. Ted said to me, "I'm not giving in to a bully. Marie will never have long-term dialysis—I'll stop it immediately."

A few days later, on a day when Ted wasn't there, Eddie showed up at the hospital accompanied by a notary and in possession of a document that awarded him medical power of attorney, durable power of attorney, and financial power of attorney, along with a quick claim deed giving him title to Marie's home and other properties. I intervened, telling the notary that Marie didn't have the cognitive capacity to understand the documents, let alone sign them.

When the notary walked out, Eddie flew into a rage and security had to remove him from the building. From that point on, he visited only when Ted wasn't there.

A few days later, as I was pulling into the parking lot to begin my afternoon rounds, Ted called.

"Eddie is stalking me, and I'm going to have to get an injunction to put a stop to it. When I got into my car this morning, he was sitting at the curb. I rolled down my window and asked him what was going on. He said he was going to follow me all day to see what I did with my time.

"Then he said, 'I want to know where you and mom got married, because I don't think you guys are husband and wife. When I prove that you're not, I'm going to get medical power of attorney, and I'll be in control. And then we're going to save my mom's life.'"

Eddie had visited his mother only twice in the last five years. Ted and Marie had been wed eight years before and he had ignored the invitation. If he had visited more often, he would have seen Ted and Marie's framed wedding certificate on their wall.

Because of Eddie's intervention, Marie was now on dialysis in the ICU, which was clearly against her expressed wishes. Twice she pulled out her dialysis catheters, either from confusion or because she was communicating what she really wanted. By now, she had been in the hospital for sixty days and wouldn't be able to go home again. At a team meeting, her nephrologist recommended she go back on permanent dialysis. This would require another procedure to place a long-term dialysis catheter.

"Is it going to make her walk again?" I asked in disbelief. "Is it going to cure her congestive heart failure? Her respiratory failure?"

He backpedaled a bit. "Well, it's going to help address her kidneys. Maybe it can help some of these other things as well."

He had opened up the can of worms. It was all Eddie needed to hear. Now I was really the bad guy, standing in the way of saving Marie.

Three days later, the kidney doctor's partner met with me.

"I talked with Ted and Eddie to make them understand that dialysis was not going to fix Marie. But we'll continue with it until we get a clear message about what the family wants to do."

Fat chance that was going to happen. And so, the deadlock continued.

I've learned the hard way that a loved one's impending death never cures family dysfunction. Quite the opposite.

In just one day, with four dying patients, I encountered every major issue that I face as a hospice doctor. Rampant denial of the inevitability of mortality. Slipshod preparation for death. Directives and MPOA documents that mean nothing. Dysfunctional relatives battling over a loved one's care. Being screamed at and threatened with lawsuits by family members. Aggressive medical treatments that only prolong a patient's suffering.

Not all days go like this, but I usually don't get called for situations where preparations have been made and patients have made their own wishes known. Emotionally, it is extremely trying. Yet, I believe passionately in what I do. Despite the confusion and chaos and occasional animosity, I've been able to change the direction of the ship just enough so that a terminally ill patient doesn't die in an institution. I help empower these patients to pick the place where they want to face life's end. I succeed in helping family members not feel responsible or guilty about a loved one's death. If I can achieve any of these goals, no matter how imperfectly, I feel I've accomplished what I'm medically and morally obligated to do. No matter how hard it is for me to go from room to room visiting dying patients and dealing with grieving families, I feel I've done my part as a palliative care doctor. The difficulty is not in talking to patients and families about death, but in being prevented from having that talk.

A couple of weeks ago, I was in the ICU when a nurse came up to me and said, "We really need you on this case. I want you to do a hospice consult. I tried to bring you in last week, but the doctor said I was being a pessimist."

I never get the easy ones. When the situation has gotten out of control, with screaming and yelling and finger-pointing and threats of litigation, they bring me in to try to fix the mess. I have to quickly find a cure for psychosocial dynamics and family dysfunction that have been around forever. It's up to me to mend all the broken fences and burned bridges, to intervene successfully in huge power struggles.

Most doctors aren't trained to deal with this kind of stuff or choose not to deal with it.

A few days ago, I was in a meeting with an intensive care doctor, one of the folks who call me only when there's nothing left he can do. He's one of those doctors who will perform any test or treatment right up to the end, no matter how hopeless the case. I was a silent participant, listening to him chat with the nurse practitioner and a couple of residents.

"Samuel is going back to the cardiac Cath Lab for more stents. If he survives, we're going to work on extubating him to see if we can get him back to rehab."

Then he looked at me and said, "We're not ready for you yet."

Not ready for me yet? Samuel had already suffered two cardiac arrests, was on a ventilator, and was scheduled to go back to the cardiac Cath Lab yet again? When would they be ready? I should have been working with Samuel's family many weeks before to come up with a plan, a realistic endpoint.

I was once asked to consult with a dying patient, but wasn't able to get to the hospital until late the following afternoon. When I arrived, the doctor had written in the patient's notes: "Palliative consult placed, still waiting for the discussion."

The patient had been in the hospital for seventy-eight days without a single discussion about his impending death, and yet I was cited for being twelve hours late to finally have that conversation. They could have called me thirty days before, or forty-five days before, or sixty days before. Not at the end, when options had been exhausted.

Once again, I was "the pessimist," the unwanted intruder, good old "Doctor Death."

And who was the ICU physician treating Samuel? "Doctor Waiting for a Miracle"? Because that's what it would have taken for Samuel to recover, leave the hospital, and resume a meaningful, functional life.

I should have been preparing Samuel's family for their loved one's end. I should have been identifying Samuel's thoughts and feelings about how he wanted to die. Instead, he went into the operating room, had surgery, and remained in the ICU. When I was finally called in to talk with the family, they said to me: "Why didn't you talk to us sooner?"

It was a question that left me speechless.

Chapter Three

You're Getting Better (But Still Dying)

I vividly remember the first time I met with a dying patient who was utterly convinced she was getting better.

"Elaine's not going to make it," her doctor told me. "You need to go tell her."

I walked into her room and introduced myself. My first step in meeting with a patient is to take a reading of what they understand about their care and prognosis. I try to look at the big picture and connect all the dots. So the first thing I asked Elaine was, "What have you been told so far by the physicians who've been seeing you? What do you understand about your disease and what you're going through?"

She was propped up against her pillow, her face pale.

"Well, I'm getting better."

"Okay, can you please explain that a little bit more?"

"Well, I came into the hospital because I was bleeding into my stomach. But the gastroenterologist did the scope, and now I'm not bleeding anymore.

"The hospital doctor said I was extremely anemic when I came in. After a couple of blood transfusions, my blood count is better now, so I'm getting better with that.

"The kidney doctor said I was in danger of kidney failure, but now my kidneys are getting enough blood and they're working again.

"The cardiologist said my heart went into this weird rhythm because of stress and anemia due to the stomach bleed. But he fixed that with medication, so my heart is better as well."

I paused to consider what Elaine had said. She addressed every reason for why she was in the hospital, except for her terminal cancer.

"Okay, I understand what these four doctors have told you. Where did you come from when you came to the hospital?"

"I was in a rehab facility."

"Why were you there?"

"Because I'm paralyzed from my waist down."

"And what caused your paralysis?"

"I have fractured vertebrae that pushed on my spinal cord and injured it. I went to rehab to learn to walk again."

Although I knew all the answers, I kept asking the questions.

"And why did your spine break?"

"Because I have colon cancer. It's spread to my liver and lungs and spine. I want to learn to walk again and then go home."

The cancer had in fact spread throughout her entire body. Elaine would never walk again, and I told her that.

"But everybody else has told me I'm getting better."

I said, "Elaine, do you understand that you're dying?"

The silence in the room was dense and lingered for some time.

"But I've had four other doctors tell me, literally in the last three hours, that I'm getting better. They sent me to the rehab center to get better."

Elaine was my first experience with "I'm getting better." Every seriously ill person wants hope. Everyone looks for anything to give them hope. An oncologist may tell a patient she has terminal cancer, but in a span of a few hours, four other doctors may tell that same patient about what they can do to help. A cardiologist will walk into a room and say, "Oh, you're getting better." I'll walk in a few minutes later and say, "You're dying."

Hope that isn't tempered by medical reality is a cruel parody of hope.

Too often, the nephrologist talks to the patient, the cardiologist talks to the wife, and the neurologist talks to Grandma, but no one provides the family with a frank and full picture of what's happening. The family is left to piece together bits and pieces of disconnected information, much of which sounds like a foreign language.

The specialty doctors speak for themselves, from their individual silos of treatment, hyper-focused on their precise areas of expertise. They're not lying to the patient and they're not being manipulative. Elaine's four doctors had indeed fixed parts of her body. They were forthcoming in their particular responsibilities, which was to fix whatever system they specialized in. Their "good news" wasn't false. They had simply failed to present the big picture.

This happens for many reasons. Crammed schedules. Fear of scaring the family. Not knowing what language to use. Doctors routinely tell me: "It's not my job to tell them, Ken. That's *your* job."

They leave it to someone else to tie it all together, to help patients like Elaine face the whole truth.

Instead of talking with each other or with the family as a whole, the sub-specialists communicate mainly through the written chart. The cardiologist comes in at 6:00 a.m., the infectious disease doctor comes in at noon, and the neurologist arrives at 6:00 p.m. By simply reading the chart, it's very difficult for everyone to get on the same page.

I've often been in a patient's room with several other doctors, each occupied with a computer.

"Oh yeah," one says, "we did this with him and now we're going to let cardiology take over and do their thing."

"We're done from an infectious disease standpoint," the other says. "We've ordered the antibiotics and will keep him on that for six weeks. I know the gastroenterologist is still trying to do a few things. We'll let him take it from there."

The cardiologist will walk in and say, "Congestive heart failure. We're going to do A, B, C, D, E, and F." The nephrologist will point out renal insufficiency. Each specialist picks his or her diagnosis and disease and goes to work.

The numbers may improve, and may look promising, but the patient is still dying.

Hospice companies are required by Medicare to have an IDT (interdisciplinary team) meeting between the various doctors treating a terminally ill patient. The purpose of the IDT is to work together as a cohesive unit to meet the physical, emotional, spiritual, and psychosocial needs of the patient and family. All members are supposed to work together as equal partners in addressing these needs. I've found these face-to-face meetings very effective in planning for end-of-life care.

These kinds of meetings are not the norm in most hospitals. Quite often, doctors aren't able to call other doctors or to meet with them face to face. Once in a while, a physician will pick up the phone and say to me, "I just saw your patient and I had some ideas about how we should go forward." But most of the time, there's so much activity going on, with doctors going from room to room and hospital to hospital, that there's little or no direct communication. Instead, each specialist records on the chart what he or she can and can't do, but there's no discussion of the big picture, of the overall needs of the patient and his or her family.

This is a huge source of frustration for me. There needs to be much better communication. A patient with a history of two cardiac arrests and little chance of recovery needs a team meeting that addresses the realities of his medical condition and his family's wishes about how his last days should be spent.

But too often, doctors don't work as a team because each specialty doctor wants to get his or her specific problem fixed as quickly as possible. Each physician stays in his or her lane. Too often, the family is told very little. And I can't be brought into the picture until the medical team requests my services. I, too, have to stay in my lane, based on the collective documentation that I get from the patient's chart or from talking with the patient's doctor.

I recently had a request for a consult with a patient who was dying from Stage 4 pancreatic cancer. I was asked to discuss his advance directives and what he wanted going forward. It was my opportunity to find out his goals and thoughts while he was still capable of communicating them.

The next day, I got a text message from the patient's oncologist canceling the consult: "This is my patient. I don't want you talking to him."

Some doctors are unsettled by the conversations I have with their patients. They feel irresponsible if they don't insert this tube or administer that drug. Some are afraid of a lawsuit if they haven't tried everything and the patient dies. I'll joke with them: "You're selling immortality. The patient is hearing that she's going to live forever if she simply takes this pill or undergoes that test."

My approach is somewhat different: "You have a finite amount of time left. We need to pick a pathway that will allow you to enjoy that time as best you can."

The patient may then decline to continue aggressive treatment and choose instead to die comfortably at home, surrounded by family. If the doctor is insisting on a different route—"We can do another test. We can do another procedure. We can give you another pill."—I'm not the best person to have in the room.

A doctor once said to me, "There are still some things I can do to this guy." Not what he could do *for* this guy or *with* this guy, but *to* this guy.

From a medical standpoint, I'm at the complete mercy of the other physicians. As a consultant, I need to be invited into the patient's care.

In certain instances, the attending physician rotates every few days to a week, leading to a new doctor taking over the case. A doctor who may have recommended stopping a certain procedure gets replaced by a new one who wants to continue aggressive treatment. This only leads to more confusion and anxiety for the patient and family. Week two rolls around, and another new doctor arrives. It's hit or miss whether any of these doctors will call me. Most end-of-life discussions take place an average of about thirty days before the patients die (NCBI research), which is not enough time to prepare for death.

At a certain point, I'll be called in for a palliative care consult. Palliative care, also called comfort care, supportive care, and symptom management, is not hospice. I don't have to be called in because the patient is taking her last breath. Rather, I can be called long before that, so we can figure out if the patient wants to be hospitalized for the sixth time, or have a feeding tube inserted, or be put on a breathing machine. I'm there to help someone manage their physical and emotional pain. The goal of palliative care is to treat, as early as possible, the symptoms and side effects of the disease and its treatment, in addition to the related psychological, social, and spiritual problems. These kinds of issues should be addressed as soon as we know that a patient has a life-limiting illness, not when he or she is on her death bed.

A palliative care patient may still want to pursue aggressive treatment and not yet be ready to transition to comfort measures. Such a patient can go home with lung disease, and I can visit her and give her medications to keep her comfortable so she doesn't have to keep going back and forth to the hospital. She can still go to see her pulmonologist. If she has trouble breathing, I'll be called to help get her through her difficulty. I can treat the patient or send over one of my team members. She can still have aggressive treatment at the hospital if she wants it.

Hospice care is a form of palliative care given to a person when treatments are no longer controlling the disease. When a person has a terminal diagnosis (usually defined as having a life expectancy of six months or less), he or she might be eligible to receive hospice care. The goal is for the patient to be treated at home, in a group home, or in an assisted living facility. Hospice patients are the sickest of the sick; by definition, they're in the dying phases of life. I'm supposed to take care of their pain, their nausea, and their vomiting and keep them from feeling they need to go someplace else to get help. If a hospice patient has difficulty breathing and goes to the hospital for treatment, then I've failed that patient.

Unfortunately, far too many patients who need palliative care don't receive it. Dr. Anil Markam of the University of

California at San Francisco studied approximately 14,000 patients admitted to long-term acute care hospitals. He found that the one-year mortality rate was high, with a little over half of older adults dying within one year. Only 1% of the patients were seen by palliative care clinicians during their stays, and only 3% were seen by geriatricians. This happens despite clear evidence that early integration of palliative care is associated with:

> "[B]etter patient quality of life, better understanding and communication about illness, improved access to home care and to emotional and spiritual supports, increased patient well-being and dignity, improved care at the time of death, and decreased symptom burden. Studies show that inpatient palliative care consultation reduces length of stay and cost per episode of care, primarily by reducing the use of necessary tests and non-beneficial treatments, and in some cases, it may prolong life." (*Palliative care: Issues in the intensive care unit in adults*, by Margaret Isaac, M.D., and Randall Curtis, M.D., MPH.)

Today, because of the opioid crisis, more and more oncologists are providing less and less pain management. As a result, oncologists, as well as other specialists, refer patients to me for that symptom management. I've got patients being referred to me to manage their pain while they're still being aggressively treated. They may or may not be hospice appropriate, but I can help them.

With these patients, it's a process of education. Have you established advance directives for your care? Has someone been given MPOA? What do you consider to be an acceptable functional status? Do you want to be treated aggressively up to the end?

I don't want to be asking these questions when the patient has a week left.

Elaine, the woman whose cancer had spread throughout her body and would never walk again, had not been asked these questions by her doctors. They did not discuss the colon cancer with her because "somebody else" was managing it. It wasn't the cardiologist's responsibility to sit with Elaine's family for an hour to discuss her colon cancer and why their loved one was not going to survive. These physicians have schedules that do not allow them that time. And, as subspecialists, they "stay in their lane," believing someone else will have the conversation. In most hospitals, you're lucky if that talk lasts fifteen minutes—if it takes place at all. According to a study by the National Center for Biotechnology Information (NCBI), less than one-third of patients and families have end-of-life discussions with their doctors.

Nine times out of ten, no one has that talk with them but me. Having that conversation, and having it in depth, is my responsibility. Exactly how to have it was something I learned on the job through much trial and error.

In Elaine's case, I had to be clear that I wasn't there to question the conclusions of the other physicians.

"I understand that one of the doctors fixed your heart rhythm. He was able to give you medication that corrected the heart rhythm that was causing your anxiety and palpitations. Now that it's fixed, you're less anxious. In that sense, you are better. Then again, we have to look at the bigger picture of what you were going through when you came here."

Now was the moment when I had to frame the big picture for Elaine as compassionately as I could.

"Even though you've been told you're getting better by four different doctors, I'm here today to tell you that you're dying. You've reached the point where the only decision you can make is where you die. So do you want to go back to the rehab facility and die there? Or do you want to go home with hospice and die with your family? This can be very empowering for someone who has lost control of her disease and independence."

Silence in the room again.

"I want to go home," she finally said. "No one put this into perspective the way you have. I've had a great life, but if I've only got a limited amount of time left, I don't want to waste it in a rehab facility. I want to be home with my family."

Within a day, she was discharged home. She died three weeks later.

In medicine today, people are "getting better" in the intensive care unit when they're dying. They're "getting better" in oncology when they're dying. They're "getting better" in all these different departments when they're dying. "Better" is a word that should never be used around terminal patients and their families.

It's my job to help them understand that while they're responding to specific treatments, their prognosis is unchanged.

I had a patient named Ruth in her late seventies or early eighties who was in the intensive care unit for congestive and renal failure. At home, she had been barely able to walk from her bedroom to the bathroom. She was declining to the point where her doctors recommended dialysis.

When I visited Ruth, I took a seat. I'm "the doctor with

the chair." Every time I have a talk with patients or family members, I'm always seated. Sometimes I'll bring a chair with me if there isn't one in the patient's room. I never stand over people. Most discussions about death (fifteen minutes at best) take place with the white-coated doctor standing at the foot of the bed, a stethoscope hanging around his or her neck.

The doctor is the authority; the patient and the family are somewhat subservient. When the doctor is standing, it implies that he or she doesn't have a lot of time. Which is probably the case—most hospital doctors have to hit their numbers, seeing twenty to twenty-five patients a day to keep their jobs. How can you have a conversation about dying when you don't have the time for it?

That's never been my approach right from the start. I've always given patients the time they needed. I'm not saying that palliative care doctors are the only people who do this. But in the medical system as it exists now, sitting down for a thirty-minute discussion is not the norm for most physicians because they're not allowed that opportunity.

When I talk about death with patients, I'm not only seated in front of them, but my phone is turned off. I'm entirely present to the moment and 100% focused on them. The person in front of me is my sole priority. I listen to what they have to say. I'm deeply respectful of the profound conversation we're about to have. In one study by *Annals of Internal Medicine*, doctors were found to let patients speak only an average of eighteen seconds before interrupting them. I don't do that. I'm there to reflect back to them what I hear them saying and to validate their hopes, fears, and concerns. The conversation is not about me.

The patient may be performing—*I'm going to fight this to the end*—but I can look into the eyes of the spouse or child and see what they're feeling. I know what they're feeling inside just by looking at them, by reading their body language and energy.

It's hard to verbalize this non-verbal communication. But when you've worked with someone a long time and developed a relationship, you can look beyond the words. You can read their anxiety and fear, whether it's their facial expressions, hand movements, or foot tapping.

I spent an hour and a half sitting with Ruth in the ICU. I reviewed her functional status and her relationship with her family. Then I said, "Do you understand what dialysis means for you? I know what your doctors are recommending, but do you understand what you'll be going through if you choose that path?" We discussed how grueling it would be—traveling to a facility for a four-hour treatment three or four times a week.

I said to Ruth, "You know that your disease is terminal, and you know that it's eventually going to take your life. Where's your quality right now going from appointment to appointment? Would it be better served spending two weeks at home with your family, rather than three or four weeks in the back seat of a car going from place to place?"

At the end of our discussion, she said, "You know what? I just want to go home and be comfortable with the time I have left."

The next day, I was in the intensive care unit standing outside Ruth's room. A nurse was speaking with her, who obviously hadn't read my note and didn't know Ruth had been visited by me. I overheard Ruth say to the nurse, "I've decided that I'm not going to do dialysis. I want to go home with hospice."

Without skipping a beat, the nurse replied, "Oh, you don't want to do that. You're young. You've got a lot of life left in you. You need to fight."

With just a few sentences, everything we had carefully worked through got turned around one hundred and eighty degrees. Having reservations about going into hospice is quite common; who wouldn't have reservations about a decision that points toward the end of life? But for a nurse to play in this cavalier way with the mind of a dying patient (and the minds of her family)? To encourage someone to fight, when fighting only meant more treatments and more suffering, with not a chance of changing the outcome?

People are in an existential crisis at the end of life. To say that they're vulnerable is a massive understatement. They're always grasping for hope. They're always latching onto that word "better." They're always looking for someone to tell them they have a reason to live. But at what point is hope oversold? At what point are the true interests of the patient overlooked? At what point are the clichés of medicine supplanting the reality of mortality?

When I'm brought in to talk to patients and their families, my role is to get them to the position where they're finally at peace with being at the end of life. Maybe not at peace with the prospect of dying, but at peace with going home to face the end with their loved ones, understanding they're going to have the resources to work through it.

And then one person—maybe a long lost relative, perhaps a well-meaning nurse—upends that hard work with their biases and agendas. *"You know what? You don't want to go into hospice. You're still young—you've got a lot of life left in you."* Who doesn't want to hear that, whether or not it's the truth?

The next afternoon, Ruth signed a consent form, had her dialysis catheter placed, and transferred out of the ICU. She remained in the hospital and dialysis was started.

About ten days later, I received a message that she wanted to talk to me again.

I sat down across from her, and she got right to the point. "I don't want to do this anymore."

And so I began helping her let go of the dialysis, assuring her it was okay to stop. Just because she started down this new path didn't mean that she couldn't reverse course. Soon she was on her way home with hospice services. She passed away within a couple of weeks with her family around her.

Angela had been in the hospital for sixty-eight days. She had a history of cancer and heart disease and came into the hospital with pneumonia and kidney problems. Her request was for full resuscitation, meaning: "Do everything that you can for me." When I came in to talk to her, she was lying in bed looking very weak.

I try to have my first hospice talk alone with a patient. With other family members not present, I have the best chance of getting the patient's true thoughts, feelings, and desires. I reviewed with Angela what she had been through.

"You have breast cancer, and you didn't make it through the entire chemotherapy because you got too sick. Now you're here because you have kidney failure, heart failure, pneumonia, and a urinary tract infection. But you're still listed as full resuscitation, so if something were to happen to you right now, you could end up on a ventilator."

Angela nodded, her eyes fixed on me.

"If so, we may have to do CPR. You might need to be shocked. If all of that happened and you end up surviving, then you'll be in the intensive care unit. Your husband has medical power of attorney. So what would you want him to do? Because if we don't talk about this, and you're in the intensive care unit for ten days, fourteen days, I'm going to have to ask him, 'Do we keep doing this? Do we put in a tracheostomy?

Do we put in a feeding tube?' If it gets to that point, what do you want?"

Angela's doctor had already been talking about once again putting a tube into her chest to drain fluid. She had had that procedure several times before due to her pneumonia.

She didn't respond, looking past me, apparently considering what I had said.

Speaking gently to her, choosing my words with care, I went on.

"Do you really want to keep doing that? Or do you want to stop, not go through anything else, and just go home and be comfortable? If so, we need your husband to clearly understand what you want done."

Angela said, "I don't want to have any more treatments in the hospital, I don't want to be on a machine, I don't want to have CPR. I want to be left alone and kept comfortable. In fact, I want to go home with hospice."

Two hours later, when I visited with her again, Barry, Angela's husband of fifty-five years, was sitting at her bedside. I began talking to him about his wife's wishes.

"Angela doesn't want to go through anything more. Not because she doesn't want to, but because she just can't. She's been in the hospital sixty-eight days. We've done everything we can. She has all these underlying conditions. Do we want her to be in the hospital for another two or three months?"

Barry said, "Well, the surgeon said that he's going to perform another procedure, and then we can send her to rehab. And this is what we want to do."

If Angela had that surgery, I knew she would end up in the ICU on a ventilator, exactly what she didn't want. And yet, her husband was telling me the opposite. The dynamics of their relationship were now dictating the situation, not Angela's stated wishes and not medical reality. Her husband was in control and in denial.

I had to be as tactful as possible in what I said next.

"With all respect, sir, you and I are not doing much but sitting next to Angela's bed. She's the one who has to go through the treatments, not us. So when you talk about 'we,' you're actually talking about you and you're making this about you."

"Well," he replied, "she wants this. She wants further treatment."

"No, sir, she told me she doesn't want that."

"Well, we'll get through this. We'll walk this path, wherever it takes us. She's a fighter. She's always been a fighter. Right, hon?"

It was a frustrating moment for me, one I had learned to navigate with patience through years of experience.

When I walk into a room to visit a dying patient, I'm not Ken Pettit. I'm a doctor. The case is not about what I want, and it can be extremely difficult to maintain that balance and objectivity. I have to understand the motivation behind someone's point of view. I'll often encounter people who have strong religious beliefs. For them, God decides when it's someone's time to die. I believe in God. I also believe that replacing our belief in God with a machine that artificially prolongs death is not appropriate.

When someone has religious beliefs different from my own, I respectfully acknowledge their views and step back. Every patient has the right to continue with aggressive treatment.

Whenever my emotions become involved, I can feel the energy change in the room. It threatens to become a confrontation, an argument. That's the last thing I want to happen, so I do everything possible to make sure the discussion is not about me. It's not about what I would do if I were in the patient's situation. Instead, I try to help them understand where they're at and what their options might be.

Someone may say to me, "When my dad put his advance directives together fifteen years ago, he told me he wanted everything done. So we're going to do everything we can medically to save him."

And my response will be: "Well, that was fifteen years ago when his functional status was 100%. But if he were plugged into a machine knowing he was never going to walk again, dress himself, feed himself, bathe himself, or clean himself after a bowel movement, would his answer still be the same today? Would he want us to do everything?"

We need to define "everything" when we're talking about treatment. Today, there is so much more technology that we can use to sustain life, but it comes with a price. If "everything" means a tracheostomy tube, would you want it? If it means a tube in your bladder or your liver or your gallbladder or your kidney, would you want it?

The list goes on and on.

If their response remains the same, that they want to do everything medically to save their loved one, then I step out of the way. The conversation is not about me. It's about what the family wants. If I go into a room and a patient's family doesn't want to change their loved one's resuscitation status, that's their right.

Some countries don't give you that right. When you hit a certain age, you're not eligible for certain procedures. They're not going to pay for a treatment costing $100,000 if the patient is not going to live another six months. In the United States, you have every right to spend every dollar to get what you want medically. That's the way the system works, and I can't change it.

But if a patient has a limited amount of time left, I try to help them take responsibility for that reality. Perhaps at no other point in their life have they ever had to take that kind of responsibility. I point out that they have the right to be selfish with their time. If they have less than six months to live, I tell them that they have the right to communicate to their loved ones how they want to spend that time. Once we establish what the patient wants, then we invite the family members back into the discussion.

I'm not taking away any pathway that could possibly help the patient. What I'm trying to do is establish a game plan where no one's suffering is needlessly prolonged.

Gently, I tried to help Angela's husband hear what I had said a moment before.

"Sir, 'we' are not going through this; she is. What do you want out of this? What is the outcome you're seeking?"

"Well, I want her to be back in the front seat of my car, sitting next to me. I want us to be able to take trips. I want to be able to do what we've always done."

What I say next is always difficult, but it has to be said.

"I'm afraid that will never happen again, based on how sick she is."

"Well, we can try the procedure the doctor recommended and then see what happens tomorrow. And if that doesn't work, we'll try something else."

"Angela's already been in the hospital for sixty-eight days, and you're telling me you want her to go through more treatments because you want her sitting next to you in your car?"

I encounter this dynamic all the time, and it's a dysfunctional one. One spouse says she wants no further treatment. The other spouse enters the picture with the opposite opinion—the doctors just need to do one more test, one more procedure, and "my wife can return to my world and be the same person she was before."

Although this is a completely human impulse, it is based on self-interest and delusion, not reality.

CHAPTER FOUR

Death Doesn't Cure Dysfunction: Why Advance Planning is Crucial

I had a patient named Rob, who was a hardcore drug addict. Only twenty-eight years old, he had shot up so many times his heart valves were infected.

    He underwent surgery to install new valves and was on long-term antibiotics, but once he came off the antibiotics, he did drugs again and got the new heart valves infected. He was on the verge of dying when I went to talk with him. His mother, who was in her forties, was seated at his bedside. His cardiovascular surgeon had seen him a couple of hours earlier and told Rob he didn't qualify for further surgery.

    "You're dying," I said to Rob. "It's only going to be a matter of time before you end up on a ventilator in the ICU. Your mother is sitting here with you right now, and she's crying. You need to give her a gift. You need to tell her what your expectations are when you decline further. If you choose to go on the machine, that's your choice and that's fine, but we know you're not going to recover. And in a little while, you're not going to be able to make your own decisions."

Rob's mother was his medical power of attorney (MPOA), but it wasn't clear what his end of life wishes were. Did he want to be in the ICU on a ventilator? Did he want CPR performed on him, even if there was little chance of saving his life?

At one conference I attended, a speaker said, "In the United States, people believe that CPR is a rite of passage to death." The procedure is routinely performed in the face of evidence that most people who have CPR don't survive the event.

Rob and his mother had never talked about these issues, nor had the doctors initiated these conversations. The other physicians either didn't have the time for that talk or got frustrated trying to have it and gave up.

Rob looked up at me and said, "I don't want to talk about it right now. Maybe later."

I waited a moment, then spoke to his mother. "Rob has the ability to make his own decisions and clearly tell you what he wants. I want this communication to happen before he gets to a point when he can no longer do so. If he doesn't make a decision now, he's going to end up on a ventilator."

I then turned to Rob. "I'm strongly encouraging you guys to have this talk because if you don't, your mother and I are going to have it when you can no longer talk about it. And that will put a huge burden on her."

Two days later, making my rounds in the hospital, I found that Rob was in the intensive care unit on a ventilator. I spoke to his mom to find out what decision he had made.

"We never had the talk," she told me. "He said it was too hard for him, so I didn't know what to do."

Two or three days later, I got a phone call from the ICU: "Rob's declining and we're not able to maintain his vital signs. Can you talk to his mom?"

The moment I walked in the room, she started crying. We spent a long time talking, and she concluded that it was time to allow him to pass naturally. He was taken off the ventilator and died shortly thereafter.

Most of the time, I'm not called in to speak with a healthy person who just got sick. Rather, I get called in to speak to an unhealthy person who just got sicker—the person with heart disease that's advancing to the point where there's nothing left to offer except a way to keep her comfortable during the final course of her life. We can bring her into the hospital, put another tube into her chest, drain out a bunch of fluids, and put her on a balloon pump in the ICU. But every medical professional involved in the case understands that this disease is not going to be cured. It's up to me to help the patient accept that understanding. It's my job to talk about the end point.

Let's say the patient has been on the ventilator for ten days. I get the call. They're talking about performing a tracheostomy and moving the temporary breathing tube in the lungs to a more permanent tube in the neck. Additionally, they want to move the temporary feeding tube from the nose and insert the tube through the abdomen into the stomach. The always hopeful doctors explain it this way: "This will be more comfortable for the patient and can be taken out when they are better."

In some instances, this is the truth, but in other cases, quite the opposite. If the patient has a severe brain injury, they will have no chance of a meaningful recovery, and we know it. I once had a doctor tell me that his training hospital had an entire floor dedicated to people with horrible brain damage and no chance for meaningful recovery. They called it the "Cabbage Patch."

So, the big question becomes: do we convert the patient from an oral tube to a tracheostomy? Or do we have Dr. Pettit talk to the patient?

When the patient was in the emergency room and having trouble breathing, the ER doctor told the family, "You know what? Let's go ahead and put this tube in her throat right now. We're going to make her comfortable, and it's only going to be a couple of days. Then we'll be able to take her off."

The family never thought about the next step because they were told it was only temporary. But no doctor can guarantee that a breathing tube is going to be temporary. In fact, no doctor can guarantee anything.

That's why it's crucial that everyone has a designated medical power of attorney (MPOA), advance directives, and other end-of-life documents in place to deal with all possible medical contingencies. (About two-thirds of Americans don't have these documents.) I shouldn't be talking to families about whether they want to make a feeding tube a long-term treatment or whether they should put their loved one on a machine when he or she will never be who they were before. These kinds of decisions should be discussed and decided years in advance.

When the family tells me, "We're going to put the feeding tube in today, and we'll cross that other bridge when we come to it," my response is: "If we're having this conversation, you're already standing on the bridge."

A family may choose to go down an aggressive treatment pathway, understanding that there's no guarantee that their loved one is going to come off a machine or survive a surgery, that all our medical knowledge and technology may not lead to a good outcome. It's their right to choose that path. But eventually, they have to face the question: what is the end point going to be?

That's why MPOAs and advance directives are so important. Completing a form in the presence of two witnesses or a notary is all it takes to appoint a healthcare proxy, but most people don't do it.

When I started out as a family practitioner, I thought an advance directive was something you put in an envelope, handed to the patient, and told them to fill out at home, to pick the person they wanted to make monumental end-of-life decisions for them, should that time come. But never did I walk people through any deep understanding of these documents and the crucial issues involved in preparing them until I was working full time with terminal patients.

Most communication about death is nonverbal. The patient is thinking, "I'm so tired. I can't keep doing this." The family member is thinking: "How much more can she take? I can't believe it's gone this far. I will never allow this to happen to me."

The patient and the family have the same feelings, but they can't communicate them to each other. They're separated by their fears and preconceptions and assumptions about death and dying. My role is to help the patient and family members verbalize what seems impossible to articulate. The patient and the family members are afraid to stop performing because they're worried they'll inflict emotional damage on each other by "giving up."

This was the bind I faced with my father. I was his medical power of attorney, not my mom. He knew I would be able to shut down the machine when necessary. My mom didn't push back against that decision, but she could never have made that decision herself. I knew it was absolutely the right decision to make, and I was fortunate that it was left on my shoulders.

When choosing your medical power of attorney, it's crucial that you pick the right person to advocate for your best interests when you can no longer do so. It's important to choose someone who will honor your wishes and not change his or her mind when the time comes to make crucial decisions.

A patient once said to me, "I don't need anything in writing. My family will know what to do when the time comes."

My response? "No, they're not going to know. Don't put that burden on them. You need to make the decision now."

I will hold the patient accountable if they try to make someone else responsible for decisions they have the ability and responsibility to make. I will work hard to guide him or her through that process. I don't want the burden to rest on someone else. The person who is dying must accept responsibility for his or her fate and not put that burden, and the potential for accompanying lifelong guilt, on someone else.

Advance directives are written documents that clearly spell out how a person wants end-of-life decisions to be made. Someone may be placed on a ventilator while being unable to make a decision about whether or not to continue that treatment. Someone may not be able to make a decision about whether a tracheostomy tube should be inserted into his neck. That's when an advance directive becomes vitally important.

One of the difficulties in today's medicine is that advance directives are usually put together by attorneys in boilerplate fashion, e.g., "If two doctors agree that I'm brain dead, then this is what I want done."

Unfortunately, with today's medication and technology, it's very hard to become literally brain dead. Therefore, advance directives have to be redefined to meet this new reality. A lot of hard questions have to be asked and answered. After a certain treatment or procedure, will I be able to carry out my most basic needs? Will I be able to feed myself, wipe my butt, take a bath or shower? Or am I going to be bedbound and reliant on medical technology for the rest of my life?

What decisions will be made based on this information?

Someone could exist in a vegetative state forever if they're plugged into a machine. We need to base advance directives on today's medicine, not on a boilerplate generated by an attorney's office. They need to address the range of reasons why people may not want their lives extended.

Even with medical power of attorney in place, I've seen disputes develop over who gets to make the final decision. Someone picks an MPOA for various personal or family reasons, but that person ends up ignoring or challenging the patient's wishes.

That's why choosing your medical power of attorney is one of the most important decisions you'll ever make. The first step is communicating your wishes to that person and all other people in the family who will be potentially involved in any end-of-life decisions.

The next step is to choose someone who will stand her ground if someone challenges the advance directive. If it's not going to be a family member, that has to be clearly spelled out. There needs to be plenty of communication to make sure that the medical power of attorney will follow your stated wishes. You need to make sure that the person is truly going to do what's best for you. If the MPOA isn't able to stand her ground in the face of pressure from family members, you're in dangerous territory.

There's always the potential for some degree of dysfunction when families are facing end-of-life decisions. In the state of Arizona, we have what's called surrogate decision-making. The state recognizes who the medical power of attorney will be if the family or patient hasn't designated that person. First in line would be the spouse, then the children, and it continues down through the family.

This creates a potential conflict if the second oldest child has been at the bedside the entire time because the father didn't want the oldest child as MPOA. That oldest child might be a person with addiction who's never been in his father's life. Yet that person now has the power to intervene at the last moment and go against the father's wishes for all the wrong reasons. That's why you must designate an MPOA who understands your wishes and who will follow them at all costs.

Arizona law says that a physician can call an ethics committee meeting with other physicians if no family member is available. If the conclusion of the committee is that the patient's resuscitation would be futile, they can change the patient's status. Nobody wants to take the pecking order that far, but that's what can happen.

When you can no longer function and you're bedbound staring into space, we can wheel you outside and point you into the sunlight every day. We can water you, make sure someone wipes your butt, and we can stick a tube in your bladder. But if that's not the life you want, you have to spell it out years before that time comes.

Again, dying patients tell me, "My family will know what I want when the time comes." But when I talk with the designated MPOA, I quite often hear the opposite: "I have no idea what he wants." Fear prevents crucial communication from taking place. In fact, there's so much fear and guilt about making end-of-life decisions that, according to one study, spouses who have the task of putting together advance directives suffer from a greater mortality rate than the critically ill patient in question.

Sometimes I'm called the "what if" doctor. Someone will say to me, "The doctor said my brother's going to be put on a ventilator for only three days, and then they're taking him off." And I'll respond, "Well, what if we can't get him off? What's the next step? What do you want to do then?"

If my options are A) live and B) die, I will almost always pick A. But if I'm terminally ill, choice A comes with consequences. If a person wants to be resuscitated, then certain steps will follow from that decision. But what if the person isn't able to make his wishes known?

It's a thousand times harder to talk about taking out a feeding tube or a ventilator tube than putting one in because it raises issues of control and guilt. It raises the issue of "pulling the plug," of "killing mom."

A decision about resuscitation should never be made in a five-minute conversation with a doctor looking at his watch, trying to fit in seeing twenty patients in a day. It just can't be done. Far too often, the only conversation that takes place is the question of whether to do CPR or to put in a feeding tube. The choice is made without much discussion or reflection, and then the doctor is off to the next patient on his list.

That kind of approach leaves a huge hole for me to try to fill. So often, I've wanted to be called in earlier so I can have an informed and in-depth discussion with the patient. I'm not going to walk in out of the blue and say to someone, "Well, you're dying." Talking about death needs to be carefully and patiently worked through over a substantial period of time.

I had a patient who tried to commit suicide on eight separate occasions, and she was constantly in and out of hospitals as a result. Ultimately, on her last attempt, she ended up in the ICU on a ventilator. She got to the point where she would never recover to a functional state. Although she didn't have an advance directive, the family agreed that she would never have wanted her life extended unnecessarily. They made the decision to compassionately remove her from the ventilator. It was the right decision, but you can't depend on people to make the right decision without an advance directive or MPOA.

It may sound like I'm against aggressive treatments for patients who are dying. That's not the case. Rather, I'm for people understanding and discussing their definitions of a life worth living. Would you want to live the way your loved one is living in the ICU? That's a question each of us has to ask ourself.

People will say to me, "They never told me what they wanted, so we have to do everything possible to help them recover."

When that happens, I lead them through a life review process.

"Let's think back. Was there ever a time your father said to you, 'If anything ever happens to me, I never want to be on a machine.'"

"You know what?" a relative will say. "When we were out to dinner one night, we were talking about my best friend's mother being stuck on a ventilator, and my father said, 'That will never happen to me.'"

I take them down a pathway that doesn't feel like they're making a decision *for* their loved one, because in my opinion, that implies control. In this situation, they don't have control. They're not imposing their wishes on their loved one. Rather, they're advocating for what the patient wants based on their loved one's values and beliefs.

I like to say I'm 95% social worker, bartender, and clergy, and 5% doctor. The medicine is the easiest part of my job.

I had another patient who was on a ventilator in the ICU for three months. The family faced the big question. The patient's mother carried the burden squarely on her shoulders:

she felt that not doing everything possible would be "pulling the plug."

I hear that expression all the time: "I pulled the plug on my mom" or "I pulled the plug on my brother." They're guilt-ridden that they caused the death of their loved one.

My role is to ease them of that guilt. After twenty-four hours of reflection, the mother of the son in the ICU agreed to let him pass naturally.

We prepare for death like we prepare for the final exam in high school or college—not until the night before. We know it's coming, but we pretend we have all the time in the world. We don't face reality until it hits us in the face.

But if you lived with the reality that your death was inevitable and might come sooner than later, you would have a different attitude toward it—whether that meant you had two more decades to live or two more weeks.

You would not be unconscious and unresponsive about death. You'd be having meaningful conversations with people who need to hear from you. You'd be making peace with your loved ones and seeking closure. If we don't give dying people the time and the support to do this, we're robbing them of a priceless opportunity.

People near the end of life need to be very selfish with their time. It's their time, not my time. The likelihood that I'm going to live far beyond them is pretty damn high. If I know I'm likely to live another thirty years, but their life expectancy is only a week, why wouldn't I let them know that so they can make the best use of the time they have left?

I was reminded of this question by Frank, a nurse in the same hospital where I practiced. We became close friends, and I also became his primary care doctor.

He went to urgent care one day because he was coughing. They took a chest x-ray and told him he had lung cancer, which was a ludicrous diagnosis to make from a simple x-ray. Naturally, Frank was incredibly upset when I saw him next, and I sought to calm him.

"There's definitely something here that needs to be addressed, but let's wait until we know what it is before overreacting. In my opinion, I don't think that's what the problem is."

In the following days, he had a CT scan of his chest. They found a spot on his lung and did a biopsy, which turned out to be negative. Frank didn't have cancer.

Two weeks later, I got a phone call early in the morning: "Ken, did you hear that Frank got killed in a motorcycle accident?"

When I went to his funeral, his family shared something with me that I've never forgotten. The false diagnosis caused Frank to take stock of his life. He made amends with people he'd been distant from and found closure. He went through the reflective process of preparing for his death. The fear that he might have cancer gave him the courage to accept his mortality and put his affairs in order, to the benefit of himself and his family. When he was killed in the motorcycle accident, he had already prepared for his death.

Frank was lucky. In the last two weeks of his life, he prepared for his end. Most of us never make those preparations. It's an opportunity we should embrace rather than turn away from.

CHAPTER FIVE ━━━━━━

Technology Makes it Hard to Die

My daughter Jodi had an extremely high-risk pregnancy and went into pre-term labor multiple times. Thanks to technology, she could monitor her contractions and download that information into her phone, where it could be immediately evaluated by a doctor. The doctor could then direct her to take medication to help with the contractions.

When I look back on Jodi's experience, it only confirms to me that our bodies are miraculous in doing what they need to do. Because of some sort of an abnormality with pregnancy, many women will miscarry when they don't even know they're pregnant. But, thanks to advances in technology, my daughter was able to avoid a miscarriage. Around her second trimester, she was in and out of the hospital to try to prevent labor.

The moment my grandson Parker was born, we knew something wasn't right. When I looked at some of Jodi's abnormal bloodwork, it struck me that her pre-term labor was her body's way of warning us. Jodi's miscarriage was trying to naturally occur, but technology prevented it from happening, and so Parker was born abnormal.

It turned out that his brain had never fully developed. He couldn't speak. He was blind and deaf. He had to get a feeding tube shortly after he was born, and before we left the hospital with him, they were talking about putting him directly into hospice. Jodi and her husband were trying to cope with this catastrophic event.

Losing a child is one thing. Having a newborn child that isn't doing well is another. How does anyone deal with that?

As a father and as a doctor, I felt helpless, much as I had felt when Steve was dying. There was absolutely no way to fix what had happened to Parker, yet I had to support my daughter and her husband in every way I could. My grandson was human, alive, and had a soul.

The doctors gave Parker additional tests, which came back negative for significant chromosomal abnormalities, and on that basis, the decision to send him to hospice was never pursued. Instead, he was sent home with Jodi to start his life. After a couple of weeks, Parker started having seizures and ended up back in the children's hospital, where tests confirmed a grossly abnormal congenital brain defect.

Jodi, Parker, and her husband lived with me and my ex-wife; we set up an intensive care unit in the house to care for him. He was in and out of the hospital multiple times, on and off the ventilator more times than I can remember.

A doctor tried to talk to my daughter about placing him in hospice. It didn't go well.

"Basically, your son has no chance," he told Jodi. "His quality of life is terrible, and continuing to drag this out is just torturing him." I understood the message he was trying to convey, but the presentation was awful.

My daughter replied, "You're fired. Get out. Never come back into his room again. I want another neurologist."

Whenever I talked with Jodi about Parker, her response never varied: "This is my son. He has the best possible quality of life given his situation, and I don't care how sick he is or how hard I have to work or what I have to put myself through. He deserves every chance he can get."

This went on for a couple of years. He was in and out of the intensive care unit and on multiple medications; he probably had a hundred seizures a day. I saw this firsthand when Jodi brought Parker to my office because she couldn't take him to a sitter.

One morning, she called me.

"Dad, Parker's got a fever. What do I do?"

"Well, call your pediatrician. They're really good about always getting you in."

That afternoon, I got a phone call from my wife screaming that Parker had gone into cardiac arrest at home. Jodi had to do CPR and call 911. They were on their way to the hospital. I called there and spoke to the emergency room doctor. It was a hospital I had practiced at long before becoming a palliative care doctor, and everybody knew me.

"My grandson is on the way over," I said. "He's got horrible congenital problems. I need you to work on him for my daughter, because if he rolls through the door, you guys do two compressions, and then you stop working on him, it's going to be devastating for her."

They got his pulse and blood pressure back. He wasn't going to die in the ER. They put him on a helicopter and flew him to the children's hospital. When I got there, I heard my daughter and her husband sobbing. Walking to the end of the hallway, I found them sitting with Parker in his room. My grandson had had another cardiac arrest in the helicopter, and as soon as they got to the ICU, the doctor said, "We need to stop this." And so they did.

Several weeks after Parker passed away, Jodi and I had a talk. I recalled that she had declined having an amniocentesis and genetic studies during her pregnancy because of the danger that the tests might cause her to have a miscarriage. The tests weren't sophisticated enough at the time to have disclosed Parker's genetic problem, but Jodi said it was a mistake not to take them anyway.

"Had I known what Parker's life was going to be and what he was going through," Jodi told me, "I would have done the tests. Obviously somebody was telling us it wasn't going to be a good thing."

What I learned from this experience was that technology had allowed Parker to be born. Jodi's body was trying to tell us what was happening, and we weren't listening. Everyone dies, but we have enough technology to make it very hard to die. Is it responsible of us to apply that technology indiscriminately, especially when we know in advance what the outcome's going to be?

Technology gave Parker three years of life, but what kind of life was it? The best life it could have been, given the circumstances, but at what cost financially, emotionally, and spiritually?

Every organ system in the body is designed to protect the brain and keep it alive. We have no machine that can take over the brain's operations. There's no USB that we can plug into the backs of our heads to keep us functioning.

But, short of that, we do have machines that can make everything else work for the most part. We have ventilators. We have dialysis machines. There's a new technology, developed in the last few years, that's called an Impella device. Inserted into your heart, it keeps the blood flowing in order to take the pressure off your heart. There's also something called a Left Ventricular Assist Device (LVAD), a pump that assists the heart until the patient can get a transplant.

So for just about every organ in the body, we now have a machine that can replace it, and we keep adding to this technology. That's what I tell patients and family members—there's always another test, there's always another tube, there's always another procedure, because we just keep coming up with this stuff. For most of human history, we didn't have this power to prolong life. Now we use this power pervasively and indiscriminately.

You can give someone another year, you can always employ a new technology, but at what functional status, what quality of life? A family may want the option of doing more tests and more procedures, but choosing that option should be an informed choice made with wide-open eyes. Too often, it's not.

Not too long ago, a pre-med student came to rotate with me. He was a very smart guy, twenty-one years old, with a degree in biomedical engineering. He was doing research on technologies to keep patients alive and had already been granted a patent for some technology he had developed.

I took him on a tour of the intensive care unit and at one point asked him, "What's your end point with the technology you're creating?"

"What do you mean?"

I said, "If you apply technology to a person in the ICU and they're discharged, you've been successful. But if 90% of the patients who receive your technology die within ninety days, what's the purpose of that technology? Do we go ahead and create it? Or do we first determine the long-term effectiveness of that technology before we put it on the market?"

At first he didn't have an answer. Then he said, "I wish you had said this to me when I was in my first year of engineering school. Then I would have had a realistic goal to work toward, rather than just fixing a problem without taking into account the end point."

Doctors are actually pretty smart people. They're scientists at heart and have the responsibility to understand and apply new scientific knowledge in their work. But at what point does that new knowledge do more harm than good?

There's almost always some sort of medication or technology that can get a patient through an acute illness. For example, there's a new technology with chemotherapy agents that uses immunotherapy to boost the patient's immune system with minimal effects. You don't lose your hair and you don't get sick to your stomach. It's a treatment that can take a few months to start working. We often know the patient only has weeks to live, yet we still give them the medication, not wanting to take away their hope and the opportunity for a miracle.

One of my patients was offered immunotherapy, but he didn't have the ability to get out of bed to receive the treatment or the time left to respond to that treatment. I told this to the man's wife.

"Yeah, I understand," she said, "but he wants to keep doing this, so I'm going to support him until he gets to the point where he can no longer make decisions for himself, and then I'm going to keep him comfortable."

A few days later, I got called to the patient's house because the family didn't know what to do. I had a meeting with them and talked about pain management because the patient had been in the emergency room three times during the previous week and his pain had not been addressed. I gave him a new pain management program that would keep him out of the ER.

The next day, the wife called. "We just had a visit at the oncologist's office. They said my husband's not ready for palliative care or hospice. They recommended more treatment, but I'm not sure what to do."

At this point, the patient wasn't responding and was getting worse. I brought him into hospice with the wife's agreement and he died five days later.

An oncologist once called me and said, "I believe my patient is going to die in less than three weeks. Please talk to the family."

When I did, they told me a different story.

"You know, we just talked to the oncologist at his office two hours ago. He said, based on statistics, that a patient in my husband's situation could live for another six months."

"Well, I really apologize, but the doctor asked me to have this meeting with you because he believes your father may only have three weeks left."

The family's response was immediate and visceral: "Why did we put him through all these procedures—chemotherapy, brain surgery, inserting a catheter into his head—if he had less than a month to live?"

I'm not questioning oncologists. They are true scientists who care deeply for their patients, but many of them promise more time to patients than they have.

You can't promise that to a dying person. We have to be honest with patients, so they can be honest with themselves.

I once asked a neurologist: "When you know a patient is dying and there's no chance of a meaningful recovery, why don't you tell the family?"

"When I walk in the room and look into their eyes," he

said, "I see that they're waiting for me to give them hope. And I can't take away that hope."

One study showed that the longer you know the patient, the more difficult it is to stop treatment and tell them their time is limited.

When a doctor doesn't feel comfortable having the necessary talk, he or she tends to intellectualize the patient's condition, and technology makes it easy to intellectualize. It becomes a discussion about blood counts or chest x-rays or the next test. It becomes a technical discussion with a farmer from Ohio who knows little about science and doesn't understand the jargon. What is left out of the discussion are the most crucial issues—what the patient wants in the little time that's left and how to best prepare for the inevitable end.

We should offer certain treatments, but at the same time also give people the choice of refusing them. We spend a lot of money doing things *to* people because they don't know that they have that right. Choice should be educated and informed, made with open eyes about the prognosis and the consequences, rather than a blind belief in the unlimited powers of technology.

Chapter Six

The Death Talk

For most of us, death is a taboo subject. Even doctors who encounter it every day can't talk about it. They're at a loss for the right choice of words. They don't know how to frame the discussion for their patients, so most of the time, it never takes place.

In medical school, I was never trained in how to talk about death with dying patients. Even with training, I don't think any physician really understands or appreciates the magnitude of these conversations until you have them. Certainly, I had no clue until I was in the intensive care unit, face to face with patients who were facing profound decisions about the time they had left on this earth.

When I was in training, one of my attending physicians told me he would never forget the first time he had to tell a patient he had cancer.

"I was a third-year medical student," he said, "in a surgical rotation. We were doing rounds. When we got to this patient's room, we reviewed the chart, and the biopsy report showed the patient had cancer. My senior resident told me to go speak to the guy and tell him the news, and the rest of the team would be in shortly to discuss his options.

"I went to the room, opened the chart, looked at his face, and told him he had cancer. The patient looked at me and asked if I was sure. I looked at his chart again and told him I was. The patient thanked me, got out of bed, and jumped out the window. We were seven floors up."

Today there are courses for medical students and doctors on how to communicate in terminal cases, but there was no such course available to me in med school. I had to learn on the job and, in doing so, I've made my share of mistakes along the way. But whenever it gets difficult to talk with someone who has Stage 4 cancer or advanced liver disease, I come back to one word—empowerment. I want to empower the patient to make the best decision.

When I'm working on end-of-life issues with a family, especially when their loved one is no longer capable of participating in the decision, I take into account their prior experiences with dying. Part of that is helping them understand how little control they have over death, something we understand intellectually but not emotionally, and that helps ease the burden of guilt.

Death shows us again and again how little control we actually have, and that lack of control leads to guilt, a huge issue when death is near. If the family decides to turn off the machine, they're accepting responsibility for the outcome. They will often say to me, "I had to pull the plug on my dad, and I've been carrying that guilt with me for the last fifteen years." They've never healed from making that end-of-life decision. They've never grieved how irrevocable that decision was. They've carried the resulting guilt for years, and now they're in the same situation all over again.

My role is to help them understand that they didn't have control over death in the past and they don't have control over it now. I don't want them to pick up a new torch of guilt to carry around for the rest of their lives. I don't want families to ever leave the hospital believing that they did something that caused the death of their loved one.

I was working with a family whose daughter Olivia had been battling breast cancer for five years. A week or so before, she had told her husband that she wasn't sure she could keep going through treatment. Olivia knew she was dying and was trying to prepare him for that.

When I walked into the room, I got the "deer in the headlights" look from Olivia's family. They weren't expecting this moment. Olivia had two children, six and eight. The six-year-old daughter was just eight months when Mom was diagnosed with breast cancer. She had never known her mom not being sick. The family had always used the word "sick" and never mentioned the cancer.

If Mom's always sick and goes into the hospital and dies, the child may, depending on their level of development, equate sickness with death. When the child's friend in kindergarten is sick, she will expect that friend to die. So I had to do developmental work with Olivia's children to explain what was happening to mom and alleviate any unreasonable fears they might have.

When a loved one is in intensive care and not likely to live through the hospitalization, I try to reword the situation for the family: "We're not going to decide what's going to happen. We don't have control in that way. Rather, we're going to make a plan based on you being your loved one's advocate. You know her better than anyone else. That's why you're here. That's why you have medical power of attorney. We need to look at what you know about your loved one and what she would want. As her advocate, you are her words and her speech because she can't advocate for herself anymore. You're not making a decision that's going to injure your loved one. You're here to advocate for what they would want."

We walk through the various options and, based on what we know about the patient, look at the next steps. They may say something like, "I know she wouldn't want to be plugged into a machine. She definitely wouldn't want a feeding tube."

A couple of days ago, I had a patient who'd been on a ventilator for four or five days. The stepdaughter had MPOA, and the patient's wishes were for full resuscitation. She said to me, "He said he wanted to fight to the end."

"We're at the end," I responded. "What else can we do? We can run one or two more tests, but other than that, we're simply throwing procedures at him to keep him going. We're doing everything we can, and he's still not recovering."

After we talked, the stepdaughter changed his resuscitation status. If he went into cardiac arrest, we wouldn't perform CPR or defibrillation. Short of CPR, we were already doing everything we could. Why put him through CPR just to say we did everything possible?

He remained on the ventilator and had another test the next day. After about two weeks on the ventilator, the talk went in the direction of a tracheostomy and feeding tube. Once again, those are not temporary things but surgical procedures with potential long-term consequences. I spoke with the family: "We've reached the point where we've done everything possible. Where do we go from here?"

Usually I'm pretty successful in connecting with and communicating difficult information to the patient and family. In many cases, the patient and family are craving the conversation. One family member told me, "We just needed somebody to tell us that she was dying. No one else said a word about it." Five doctors had treated the patient and said the prognosis was poor, but they never communicated much beyond that.

What did they talk about with the family? What, if anything, was explained to them? How much did the oncologist talk to them about side effects before the treatment? In defending the treatment, the provider will often say, "They signed the consent form." But then I'll talk to patients who've had chemotherapy and are feeling horrible: "If I knew what the side effects were going to be, I never would have done this." If the patient was told about the side effects, how much did they actually hear? Was she caught in the mindset of believing that the chemo would save her life?

A patient may be awake, alert, and talking to me in a totally clear-minded way, yet he's still dying. When I talked with one such patient about going to hospice, I got a very strong reaction. So much of my work revolves around alleviating people's fears and misconceptions about dying.

"When my father went into hospice," he said, "all they did was give him morphine and Ativan, and then he died. And now you're telling me I need to do the same thing? I don't want morphine, I don't want Ativan, and I'm not going to die."

"Do you really want to be in this hospital?"

"No."

"Well, we can give you services at home, so if you have chest pain or difficulty breathing, we can alleviate your pain. But we're not going to pump you up with any unnecessary drugs."

I had a patient who was going to dialysis three days a week only because he had been told that's what he had to do. I assured him that this wasn't the case.

"Well, I was told if I don't go, I'll die a miserable death."

"You're not going to die a miserable death," I told him. "It's my job to make sure that doesn't happen. You'll be comfortable. Do you still want to continue to go through dialysis?"

He said, "I wear a hat to dialysis that says 'Walking Dead.' We sit in a room looking at each other. The next thing you know, the person that's been in the chair alongside me for two years is gone. A new person comes in to fill the empty chair. I don't want to do this anymore."

I do everything I can to let people know that they can be comfortable. A hospice patient may say to me, "I want to die," but that person doesn't want to commit suicide. They just don't want to go through whatever pain they're going through.

"Why do you want to die?" I'll ask.

"Because I still have this horrible pain."

This is an opportunity to educate patients about pain management, a crucial aspect of the work I do.

"I can treat your horrible pain," I'll say. "I want to give you as much quality time as you can possibly have. I don't want you to spend the last days of your life wishing you were dead because you're in pain."

In hospice, we manage medications to make people as comfortable as possible. We manage symptoms of death—difficulty breathing, chest pain, nausea, etc. We manage their psychosocial and spiritual needs. We enable people to pass comfortably without experiencing painful symptoms.

Medicating a dying patient is a careful balancing act. We don't want to rob patients of quality time. Drugs for pain and anxiety can have multiple side effects, such as fatigue and altered awareness. Someone who is very tired can fall and break a hip. Other patients will drift off to sleep, which at times can rob them of interactive time with their families.

If I can give the patient a drug that manages their symptoms with minimal sedation, they can be awake and alert and interact with their families. Then I believe I've done what I'm supposed to do. Have I stopped the disease? No. But I've given the patient the gift of quality time.

Usually, when pain management is framed that way, resistance softens. The patient realizes that calling 911 is a terrible resource when other more humane options are available.

When some physicians don't feel comfortable talking about mortality, they intellectualize the subject. They'll say the white cell count is getting better, or the creatinine is improving, or the pH is this or that, but what does that mean to the average person? Such language prevents effective communication about death.

The cardiologist will write down on the chart that the patient's ejection fraction is such and such. When I go in and talk to the patient, he has a terrified look. *What do you mean I've got a bad heart?* The physician has talked to him about his ejection fraction or aortic stenosis or cardiac output or whatever, but how is that information perceived and understood by the patient?

Doctors may focus on medical markers because that's what they're trained to do. But if you're not a medical professional, being told "the ejection fraction is 30%" means nothing.

One patient greeted me by asking, "Dr. Pettit, what's my white cell count?"

My question to him was, "What does the white cell count mean to you?"

"Well, the other doctor said my white cell count is getting better."

The patient became focused on an isolated piece of information that he didn't understand in order to grasp the hope that he was getting better. But a white cell count can be improving while the patient is still dying. By intellectualizing the prospect of death in the language we use, too many doctors are forestalling the patient's ability to make peace with mortality and prepare for it comfortably.

We need to be honest with them. Maybe they want to take one last trip to Yosemite, heal a family rift, or meet their newborn grandchild. They shouldn't be denied that opportunity. If they're not going to live much longer, based on medical realities, they should be told that, clearly and directly, in language they understand. Over and over again, I've found that patients and families crave this information.

I had a patient who was clearly dying of liver failure. The doctor told the family that everything possible had been tried but wasn't working. The patient still wanted everything possible to be done. I went in to talk with the family.

"What do you understand about what the physicians have told you?"

"Well, he's not doing well, but there are things that we can still do."

"I want you to understand that he's dying."

There was silence in the room. The patient's head went down in submission. Several family members shook their heads and started to cry.

"We needed to hear that," the man's brother said to me. "All we needed to know was that he was dying."

Hearing that word got them to a place where they could face the reality of the situation and prepare for it.

I went to visit a forty-eight-year-old woman with liver failure. "I think you've got about a week to live," I told her. "We can keep you alive for two weeks, maybe three weeks, with technology and medication. But if we don't do anything, I believe that you're going to die in a week or less. Given that information, what do you want to do with the rest of your life?"

She looked me straight in the face and said, "Your job sucks. You have to tell people the unvarnished truth." Then she gave me a big hug.

"I want to talk to my son," she went on. "I haven't seen him in a while and I need to connect." She made a couple of phone calls, went home, and had a meeting with him. They talked about all the long-postponed things they needed to talk about.

She died four days later, but in that time, she healed her relationship with her child. She was able to find words for the feelings she had held in for so long. Before we talked, she hadn't even thought about reaching out to him.

When I visit with a terminal patient and her family, my beliefs are out of the picture. I'm not trying to steer the talk one way or the other. I'm merely providing them with information. I provide these options without bias, almost generically.

First, I'm going to look at the patient's gender, age, and ethnic background. If possible, I need to know her religious beliefs. What is the patient's education level? Are there dysfunctional patterns within the family? Who has medical power of attorney? Which family member is going to yell the loudest and possibly go against the patient's wishes? Who's going to act out of guilt rather than out of compassion for the patient's best interests? Will a son who hasn't seen his father in fifteen years suddenly show up and scream at the MPOA about what needs to be done? Will he interfere with the transition to hospice, and then get on a plane and fly out of town, released from the guilt at having been estranged from Dad?

This is the kind of information I put in the patient's chart. It's not just about the person's blood pressure and white cell count. It's not just about what's going on medically. Even more crucial are all the psychosocial factors that affect a patient's care—or that should affect it. Is the family no longer able to provide care at home? Do they need help with funeral arrangements? Do they need assistance from a chaplain?

After these psychosocial dynamics have been addressed, I turn to the medical needs of the patient.

Patients commonly ask me, "If this was your mother, what would you do?" I give them my honest response: "It's not my responsibility to answer in those terms. What I may or may not do with my parents can be totally different from what you may or may not do with yours." I put it back on them and say, "This is *your* family member. What are your beliefs and values that affect what we should do at this point?" Once it's been framed that way, I try to give them some unbiased options. The language I use keeps me out of the picture.

This is particularly true when it comes to religion and spiritual beliefs. Religions vary widely in how they approach death and dying and in the kinds of rituals that are acceptable. Muslims and Buddhists may have completely different ways of approaching this issue. When religious beliefs come up, I have to be open and accepting about the patient's views and respect the fact that their religion has been a major influence throughout their entire lives. Their values and beliefs are formed by that filter, not by my experiences.

Because of their religious beliefs, one family wanted every last medical treatment to be tried. "If we don't do everything possible," the wife told me, "then in our view, my husband is committing suicide."

At this point, he was suffering from such severe bone pain that it literally took him two hours to get from his bed to a gurney to be transported to the dialysis center. He said he wanted to stop treatment and pass comfortably at home with his family around him, but because of his religion, he felt he couldn't make that choice. I later heard that he died in a health center while receiving dialysis.

I don't believe someone is committing suicide by forgoing needless treatments, but I have to put myself in the shoes of those who hold that belief. As frustrating as that situation might be for me personally, all I can do is give the patient information and options.

Another religious belief I have to contend with is the power of divine intervention. Many patients are waiting for it to happen, and until it does, they're going to continue down the aggressive pathway. They believe in miracles and trust God, but at the same time, they're not going to take away that piece of technology that's keeping their husband or daughter alive. They'll say to me, "I want my family member to die a natural death." Yet they don't let that happen, and for many religious people, this is not a contradiction.

"They've been trying to die a natural death," I'll say, trying to open up a discussion, "and we won't get out of the way. We've got all this equipment that's keeping them alive."

"We're not in the way," is the typical response. "We're using technology because God gave us the intelligence to create it. God gave us the skill to develop the feeding tube, and he gave you the ability to use it."

If a patient has a religious belief, I obviously have to respect that, even if the path they're going down is, in my view, not the best one. If someone is adamant about fighting to the end, I can't force my opinion on them. I can't go into that discussion with my personal biases and talk to people about what *should* happen. If I'm a Catholic and you're a Mormon, that difference goes out the window because the discussion is not about me. I can only try to rephrase or reframe my views.

"We're putting this in God's hands," they'll say.

"Well, God's been trying to work with him for weeks here," I'll say gently, "and we keep getting in the way. It may be in God's hands, but we're not letting Him do his work."

When someone is terminally ill and actively dying but fighting to the end, I return to the patient's motivations. Do they keep fighting because they're afraid of dying? Out of religious belief? Because they're performing for the family? What is the basis for their attitude?

If someone is very set in their thinking, she can become very hard to work with. In that case, I will take a step back and return periodically to talk with her. Over the course of time, when she realizes that she's running out of options and time, I can come back around and see if her views have changed. It's a gentle process that can't be forced.

When the long-estranged brother shows up and goes against the patient's wishes, I also have to deal with him in a way that's non-judgmental and non-confrontational. I have to understand where he's coming from, whether it's guilt or a deep-seated family dynamic over which I have no control. I have to keep my emotions in check. I have to maintain a positive energy. If I speak in an uncomfortable or angry way, those emotions will be reflected back to me by the family.

At the same time, the meddling relative needs to be told the ground rules in a calm, clear, and fair way.

"I want you to be aware that your father is dying, and he's chosen to be comfortable. He's chosen to work with hospice. I'm letting you know so you can have the opportunity to see him before he dies. You know that a plan has been put in place by the other family members. If you can't honor that plan, it might be better to wait to visit until you can accept it. I can help you understand his decision. The focus right now is on Dad and making him as comfortable as possible."

I met recently with the son of a very sick man who didn't want to be on a machine. The son had a contrary opinion.

"I want to keep him alive," he told me, "until he either wakes up and tells me he doesn't want to do this anymore, or until he dies of his disease."

"What if he ends up on a machine? He doesn't want that."

"If that happens, it's only going to be for a week."

"Didn't we talk about what happens if he has a tracheostomy and we put in a feeding tube? What are we going to do from that point on?"

"Well, at that point, I'll put a stop to it."

I worked with him gently to point out the inconsistency of what he was telling me.

"You're telling me you will honor your dad's wishes by not allowing a tracheostomy and a feeding tube, but until then, you're going to allow him to be on a machine? Do you understand the confusion that I'm having here? Your father is likely to end up on a ventilator. That's what's coming, and he's not going to get off of it. Why shouldn't the end point be *before* we have to apply these technologies to keep him alive, not after?"

It's always a delicate dance to make sure someone understands that no more can be done. Selfish is a hard word to use with people. Someone will say to me, "I don't know what I'm going to do. We used to do so many things together."

When I'm working with primary caregivers for people with chronic illnesses, I help them process the undeniable fact that losing their loved one is going to create a huge hole. They may be losing not only their spouse, but their entire purpose in life: "What am I going to do when my wife dies? I've been taking care of her for the past fifteen years."

And then I'll say, "I know you're going to have a big hole in your world when she passes. You're losing your identity because it was always tied to her. We need to work on your grief to help you understand her death cannot be prevented or controlled."

When families decide that they want to transition from aggressive treatment to comfort treatment and allow the natural course of death to occur, they will sometimes set a time: "We're going to take Uncle Dave off the machine at 6:00." When I walk into his room at that time, everyone is staring at the clock. I will then cover it up because the end of life is not a death sentence. I don't want them to focus on an arbitrary deadline. I don't want them to stare at a machine. I want them to focus on the person and his passing.

It's the same in the ICU—I don't want the family staring at monitors on the wall. I shut them off. The alarms get turned off. I don't want them waiting for a monitor to flat line. I want them to be entirely focused on their loved one.

When death is near, I have to educate families about the signs and symptoms that are non-verbal. If the patient is asleep and totally non-verbal but is breathing forty times a minute, that person is not comfortable and needs medication in order to relax enough to pass away.

It's hard to die when you're uncomfortable. You've got all of those physiological things happening to your body. You're agitated, you're in fight or flight mode, and you've got that terminal restlessness where you can't sit or lie down.

Even nurses have to be educated. Some of them are wary

about giving too much medication at the end. But medication does not hasten the death of anyone. This is not physician-assisted suicide. This is not giving someone an overdose. Medication gives people the ability to be comfortable while it plays out, without guilt or regret. This discussion is also part of "the death talk."

We don't have control over death, but we do have control over how we choose to talk about it when it finally comes.

CHAPTER SEVEN

The Money Game (or You're Not Dying Fast Enough)

When someone who's potentially terminal goes into a hospital and the doctors do everything to try to save that life, there's not a whole lot of discussion about money. A single chemotherapy infusion can cost an insurance company or Medicare as much as $15,000, but no one talks about that. As long as insurance is in place, you can charge whatever you want. It's an open ticket when it comes to keeping someone alive. Put a patient on a ventilator, do dialysis a couple of times, give them expensive medication to control blood pressure, and you can easily burn through $100,000 in a week or so. I had a patient who came into hospice with prostate cancer. He took three pills a day at a cost of $12,500 per month. He was dying from his cancer yet still taking his pills.

Of course, it's not just terminal patients who pay high prices. The U.S. has long had the highest costs in the world for healthcare.

According to *The New York Times* (Dec. 27, 2019), for a typical angioplasty, a procedure that opens a blocked blood vessel to the heart, the average U.S. price is $32,200, compared with $6,400 in the Netherlands or $7,400 in Switzerland. A typical M.R.I. scan costs $1,420 in the United States, but around $450 in Britain. An injection of Herceptin, an important breast cancer treatment, costs $211 in the United States, compared with $44 in South Africa.

Spending on the elderly and seriously ill is an enormous part of this money pile. An incredibly small group of patients (about 5%)—the "super-utilizers" or chronically ill patients who repeatedly return to hospitals—accounts for half of all health care spending (*The New York Times*, Jan. 8, 2020). About 25% of all Medicare spending is spent on people in their last year of life. Yet studies have shown that the less money spent in that last year on medical interventions, the better the death experience for patients and their families (Archives of Internal Medicine).

Oncologists are the true scientists in the field of medicine. They have to keep up on everything because there's so much going on in cancer research. They know when a patient's not going to survive, and yet they will still tell me, "It's up to the patient to say whether or not they want to continue to do this. I don't want to take away their hope."

The patient has a 5% chance of surviving twelve to eighteen months. Everyone wants to believe they're in that 5%.

A patient may get chemotherapy but end up in the hospital two days later, getting multiple treatments for the next two weeks to get their kidneys, bone marrow, and heart working again. Then they're "healthy enough" to resume chemotherapy. Two days later, they're back in the hospital for more treatments and die a short time later. The doctors knew the patient was terminal, but they didn't want to take away hope.

We need to reframe what hope means in the medical profession. There's a difference between hope and miracles.

We can hope that someone who's terminal isn't led to believe that they're going to live. We can hope that someone has a high quality of life in their last four to six weeks. We can hope that someone doesn't die a miserable death. These are realistic hopes, and they cost a lot less than unrealistic ones.

Some published studies have shown that certain cancer patients in hospice and palliative care programs have a life expectancy of about two and a half months longer than cancer patients receiving chemotherapy treatments. That's because their quality of life and functional status are better, and we're spending far less money to give them that benefit.

If a physician continues to offer treatments while knowing that a patient is not going to survive, shouldn't that doctor face some sort of financial liability? If a patient was subjected to expensive treatments near the end of life and still died within a month, and the attending doctor was responsible for paying back the cost of those treatments, would physicians be more honest about giving people "hope?"

How many families would put their credit cards on file to pay for treatments that do little to extend the lives of their loved ones? The same logic should be applied to doctors. Everything changes when there's a financial liability.

Today I am going to the ICU to see a patient who's been on a ventilator for two days. Based on the patient's wishes, he should not have been put on the machine. Unfortunately, when he was in crisis, having trouble breathing, he was told that only a machine would keep him comfortable, and without it he would die. Physicians should be able to honor a patient's wishes. They should be prepared to provide them with the comfort they need when they transition to the dying process.

But some physicians continue to offer aggressive treatment because they get caught up in the dynamic of one more test or one more tube. Each of these treatments comes at an incredible cost, physically, emotionally, and financially. Physicians have the ability to say no: "Your bone marrow is failing, your kidneys are failing, your heart is failing, and your functional status has declined to the point where you are no longer able to get out of bed or walk to the bathroom. We can do more, but should we?"

There is always a way to justify the next test, tube, or treatment. But there are also things we can offer that can relieve the suffering. Give the patient and family the time they need to prepare for death. Give them options. Help them meet their physical, psychological, and spiritual needs. Let them find peace with death.

And save the system a hell of a lot of money in the process.

One example of an expensive life-prolonging treatment that has little to do with a patient's quality of life is the implantable defibrillator, which restores a normal heartbeat by sending an electric pulse or shock to the heart. They are used to prevent or correct an arrhythmia, a heartbeat that is too fast or irregular. Defibrillators can also restore the heart's beating if the heart suddenly stops. Patients have to meet very specific criteria to receive one. Their hearts have to be so sick that they're in danger of going into a fatal rhythm.

The device itself costs about $25,000. Add the surgical procedure to implant it as well as monthly monitoring, and the bill for the first year can top $50,000. And yet, this device does absolutely nothing to improve one's quality of life.

The person who will benefit from an implantable defibrillator is a healthy and functional person who has had a heart attack or other cardiac event. It's not an eighty-five-year-old who is chair-bound from chronic congestive heart failure, diabetes, hypertension, and COPD, and who has been repeatedly hospitalized. Those are the same criteria for admitting someone to hospice, and yet we instead choose technology to treat them. Quite often, no one talks with that eighty-five-year-old about other options before the devices are implanted.

Doctors will tell such a patient: "If your defibrillator shocks you, it means it saved your life." Ironically, this can increase the patient's fear of mortality. Had it not gone off, they would be dead. Every moment going forward, they're reflecting on that stark fact. Some patients experience severe PTSD because of the fear of being shocked again.

A Web MD article from February 2017 stated that 38% of those who are shocked by the device did not actually need it in the first place. And remember the cost—$25,000.

Very ill patients will get the defibrillator and go home briefly, only to experience readmission after readmission to the hospital for congestive heart failure. Only then do I get the call, "Hey, he's been admitted four times in the last four months. Maybe you need to go talk to him." Maybe I should have had the opportunity to talk to him before he received the device.

Approximately 25% of the patients admitted to hospice with implantable defibrillators will get shocked at least once. I try to have my patients understand that the defibrillator only prolongs the dying process and causes needless suffering. I encourage them to deactivate the device. I'll say to a patient: "Do you want the device to keep you artificially alive? Or do you want to let nature take its course?"

I had a patient choose to keep the defibrillator on. One night, I was called by my triage nurse because the patient had been shocked multiple times. During the call, I heard him in the background, yelling for it to be turned off.

I had a ninety-two-year-old patient who resided in an assisted living facility because he had dementia. He couldn't feed or bathe himself and had a hard time moving from his bed to a chair. One day, he took a couple of steps down the hallway with his walker, and his defibrillator went off, saving him from a potentially fatal heart rhythm but shocking him so hard that he fell backwards and broke his neck, paralyzing him from the neck down. He had to be intubated and placed on a ventilator in the hospital's trauma center. Without it, he couldn't survive. Guess who got a call to talk to the family about turning off the ventilator and defibrillator?

If the physician was financially responsible for such a treatment, would he or she think twice about recommending it?

The opioid crisis was the result of physicians across the country prescribing pain medicine in excess. With the stroke of a pen, the SUPPORT Act of 2018 changed that. Physicians were told that if they continued to over-prescribe opiates, they would be subject to sanctions and could potentially lose their licenses. Overnight, the use of opioid medication in the U.S. was drastically diminished.

But physicians treating terminal illnesses in the U.S. mostly have a blank check. You can do whatever you want unless the government says you can't. That's not the case in other countries.

In Canada, fewer than 7% of patients over eighty-five receive dialysis. The number is less than 5% in Australia and New Zealand. By contrast, in the United States, a study found that more than 40% of VA patients with advanced kidney disease receive dialysis. Some patients have actually had their competence challenged when they decline dialysis to opt for more conservative care.

If doctors want to prolong life, no matter how pointlessly, the gloves are off with absolutely no expense spared. They're going to treat you until the moment of your last breath. But that's not the case when you're in hospice and actively dying. In fact,

Medicare's guidelines financially penalize hospice companies if their patients live too long.

To qualify for Medicare's hospice benefits, a patient needs to have a disease that a physician determines to be terminal, with the likelihood that the patient will die within six months if the disease is allowed to run its natural course. Therefore, in recommending that someone go into hospice, a physician has to accurately predict how long that person will live based on the information they have about the patient's cancer, heart disease, lung disease, kidney disease, etc.

What services are provided with the six-month hospice benefit?

- A physician on call 24 hours a day, seven days a week, who is responsible for providing solutions to your problems, not sending them back to the hospital.
- An RN case manager who visits you as many times a week as needed by the progression of your disease.
- A nurse on call 24 hours a day, seven days a week, to handle any unforeseen issues.
- A certified nursing assistant to help you with your increased needs of self-care, bathing, shaving, brushing your teeth, etc.
- A social worker to help with your psychosocial needs, including funeral planning, placement in a group facility if you can no longer live alone, meals, counseling, etc.
- A chaplain for spiritual needs.
- Bereavement counselors.
- A respite stay if your family needs a break and inpatient services for symptoms that cannot be managed at home.

- A volunteer to spend time with those who otherwise have no one to talk with.

All of these services, over a six-month period of time, cost less than an implantable defibrillator, a cycle of chemotherapy, or a week in the intensive care unit.

But if a patient admitted to hospice lives longer than six months, Medicare can penalize the hospice company by billing it for all the services provided to the patient past that time. A patient living beyond Medicare's prescribed benefit period may make the hospice subject to financial liability for that care. Chemotherapy treatments can cost hundreds of thousands of dollars per person, a blank check, and no one questions it.

Sound insane? It gets worse.

If I have an extremely ill patient who is not declining and deemed custodial (living beyond the six months), I have to discharge the patient to avoid a potential Medicare liability. I have to send the patient back into the community for what's called an "extended prognosis." These patients may reside in a group home. Some may be at home. Some of them are bedbound, can't speak, and don't eat or drink on their own, but group home medical staff or family members continue to drip enough nutrition into their mouths to keep their bodies functioning. It can take a very long time to die, even if you're getting the minimal amount of nutrients.

Quite often, the group home or family member will contact a different hospice company because they feel their dying loved one has been dumped into their hands. The new hospice physician arrives to see a bedbound patient who's getting nutrition through a syringe, looks cachectic (her muscles are wasting away), doesn't speak anymore, and is incontinent. Based on what this new doctor sees, he or she determines that the patient has less than six months to live, and the patient is readmitted to the new hospice company. Because of this readmission, Medicare guidelines can make the previous company liable for the patient's treatment, even though someone else has taken over that patient's care. And I have no control over that patient's care or how long they're in hospice.

In fact, if someone is in hospice for just sixty days (well under the one hundred and eighty day limit), Medicare calls that "a long length of stay," which leads to increased scrutiny and a possible audit of that company.

If audited, they receive a friendly message: "Why are your patients living so long? One of them was declining for three months, and then all of a sudden, at four months he didn't have any weight loss, chest pain, or shortness of breath. You should have discharged him at Month Number Three. Your medical director obviously doesn't know what he's doing."

Medicare concludes that I suck at my job because I didn't accurately predict the patient's mortality, not exactly an easy thing to do.

Researchers at Stanford University have explored using AI (artificial intelligence) to predict someone's death with greater accuracy, which can help doctors steer patients toward palliative or hospice care much earlier. The Stanford researchers found that they needed to take into consideration 900 different data points to be able to predict death with any degree of accuracy.

That's the standard I'm being held accountable to by Medicare—taking into account nearly a thousand pieces of data to predict the date of someone's demise.

The Stanford researchers acknowledged that three months is the minimum amount of time needed to prepare for one's death. If AI can predict someone's death with greater accuracy, we can give patients and families more time to prepare and not subject them to futile treatment. Right now, people come into hospice so late that the average length of stay for a patient in hospice was about eighty-nine days in 2018, not long enough to get its full benefits. According to the National Hospice and Palliative Care Organization, the median length of stay in hospice care in the U.S. is only eighteen days, which has changed little in the last fifteen years (NHPCO, Aug. 2020). Yet Medicare considers sixty days to be too long a stay.

The number one complaint families have about hospice is that their loved ones didn't enter it sooner (U.S. Centers for Medicare & Medicaid Services). In fact, because of the way our medical establishment works, most people coming into hospice from a hospital die within just thirty days.

This is the Catch-22 I have to deal with every day—people aren't spending enough time in hospice to reap its benefits because physicians don't want to under-promise "hope" to patients or their families. Yet if they live too long in hospice, hospice companies are penalized.

When this happens, it leads to Medicare's second conclusion about hospice—I'm intentionally milking the system and committing fraud, which puts me into a potential criminal liability. I can lose my Medicare number, face a hefty fine, or, in the worst-case scenario, be put in jail.

Shouldn't the liability be spread all around the healthcare system in a more equitable way? Shouldn't it also apply to an orthopedic surgeon who does knee surgery on a poorly-functional eighty-five-year-old, or an ICU doctor who treats a patient aggressively in her last week of life, or a doctor who does dialysis on a ninety-two-year-old? None of them are penalized, because, in the eyes of the medical establishment, and society as a whole, these doctors are doing the right thing. We're willing to pay $100,000 to treat patients who will die in a week, but we're not willing to give any slack to doctors who are trying to compassionately treat dying patients in their last days.

If we're directing money and resources toward artificially preserving life rather than helping families navigate the realities of dying, then our priorities are disastrously misguided.

Chapter Eight

How to Make Doctors Work for You

My mom and dad were attached at the hip. The two of them sat side by side in recliners for years, laughing and cussing and watching TV. They were entirely dependent on one another.

Mom was dad's primary caregiver when he was sick; when he died, it left a gaping hole in her world. She suffered from horrific post-grief depression. Fortunately, because of my work, I had the training and resources to help her. I spoke with one of my bereavement counselors and asked her to spend some time with my mom.

She worked very, very hard to process her grief, and after a few years, Mom no longer needed intense counseling. She started attending events again and appreciating the milestones of the grandkids. Whenever I walked in with them, she would say to me, "If your father was here, he would love this."

"Of course he would, mom, but he would also want you to enjoy your time going forward, honoring his life and legacy the two of you created."

One morning she woke up and couldn't speak, paralyzed on one side from a devastating stroke. She ended up in the

ICU. As with many stroke victims, she had problems with aspiration; food got into her lungs every time she swallowed. The recommendation was that she get a feeding tube; otherwise, as explained to me, she would die of pneumonia.

Mom's response was immediate and unwavering: "Absolutely not." She knew the deal. She had been a nurse for years, in addition to being dad's primary caregiver. She chose to live on her terms, not by the recommendations of doctors.

The stroke affected her speech, and my mom loved to talk more than I do. It felt like a horrible trick had been played on her. She was able to walk a little bit, but her dominant side was useless.

Whenever I asked her a question, her response would be, "Yes, yes, yes, yes, yes." If she wanted to say "Tuesday," it might come out as "Purple." She had expressive aphasia. She knew what she wanted to say but couldn't say it. Because her dominant hand was paralyzed, she lost her ability to write, a skill only partially regained after countless hours of physical therapy.

Because she didn't have the feeding tube, she developed pneumonia soon after her stroke and ended up back in the hospital. She never got to a point where she needed to be put on a ventilator, but she was sent to a skilled facility for rehabilitation. That was in 2014. Ever since, it's been a revolving door for her, going in and out of the hospital.

This is the woman who was totally dependent on my father, who had horrific post-grief depression, who arduously worked her way back through that. And now, suffering from the effects of her stroke, she has chosen to live on her own terms.

I use this experience when I work with families of stroke victims or the terminally ill. Their loved ones have potentially lost their entire independence. They have significant deficits. Maybe one of the few sources of joy left to them is eating ice cream, but that simple joy could lead to aspiration, pneumonia, and death. What choice do you make then, especially when mom's never going to be able to live independently anymore?

My mom chose her own pathway. She empowered herself. She was willing to take the risk of not having a feeding tube because she wanted to continue to eat comfortably. But eating comfortably raises the risk of aspirating. And some people who have never even had a stroke aspirate their food and end up dying.

This is the complexity of choices facing terminal patients, choices usually presented in ways that don't allow people a wide range of options. If you're told you're going to choke to death without a feeding tube, what choice would you make?

A more compassionate way of speaking would be to say: "You don't have to have the feeding tube. Yes, you're at greater risk when eating. You could aspirate, get things into your lungs, develop pneumonia, and die, but you're going to be able to drink your beer and eat your pizza all you want."

There are always ways to help that person take nourishment by making some adjustments. Avoiding invasive treatments when you don't need them is another form of empowerment. And the foundation of empowerment is to ask questions of your doctors so you can make an informed choice.

The vast majority of people are intimidated by doctors or, if not intimidated, don't know how to question their treatment. Without asking questions, there can be no empowerment.

A large part of my job is educating patients that they don't work for their doctors. Instead, the doctors work for them. Patients need to understand that it's okay to question what a doctor is telling you, that the doctor's advice may be the textbook advice but may not always be in YOUR best interest. To make doctors work for you and not vice versa, you have to be knowledgeable enough to ask questions.

Older generations gave wide deference to doctors. They were more likely to follow their recommendations than pursue an alternative path. They were less likely to question their treatment. That attitude is changing, and needs to change.

A large part of the problem, as this book has shown, is that the options doctors recommend are not presented in the most helpful ways. Telling someone "we can do this procedure or you can die" is not a great option when you're having trouble breathing or experiencing chest pain. Even younger physicians tend to present options as "do or die." That's how the system works, and patients get caught up in that system.

I had a patient whose status was "do not resuscitate, do not intubate." He got into a medical crisis and was having trouble breathing. The ICU doctor told him: "If I don't put you on a machine, you're going to die. But if I do, then you're going to be able to breathe easier."

When this patient was of sound mind and body, he had already made the decision not to be on a machine. Now he was being told he had to do so in order not to die a miserable death. If a doctor doesn't use appropriate language to discuss alternative options for comfort—options that don't require being on a machine—that's an ethical lapse in my view. Especially when the patient's stated wishes are being willfully disregarded.

As stated earlier, I worked as a primary care physician prior to transitioning to palliative care. One day, I was in the doctor's lounge talking with another physician about communication. He looked at me and said, "I really have to tell you, I hate your patients."

I was taken aback. "Whoa, what do you mean?"

"Your patients come to me with a list of questions. It destroys my entire schedule. One question leads to another question, and the fifteen-minute appointment becomes a forty-five-minute one. It's easier for me to take care of five much less informed patients, where I can go in and smile, pat them on the head, shake their hands, and get out of there in five minutes so I can see my next patient."

Guess what? I never sent that doctor another patient of mine. I'll never put a time limit on answering questions from patients.

In my opinion, the more technical or intellectual the physician is in presenting information, the less likely the patient will challenge that information. People are disinclined to challenge authority, especially when it's backed up by scientific and medical terms beyond their grasp. Some doctors may see the only option a patient has to continue to live is to place them on a machine, not talking about keeping them off. They don't know how to have that discussion.

Unless you say, "I don't want this" or "I want another option," you can end up signing consent forms for this and that, and you lose control of your care—even if you have an advance directive in place that clearly states your wishes.

We need to make sure we understand that, as consumers of healthcare, doctors work for us. We need to ask questions. If there are other options, including conservative management, doctors need to talk about those options. Or bring in someone like me to discuss them. If options are presented as either/or—"Either I can perform bypass surgery on you or you can die"—it forecloses the ability of people to make nuanced decisions.

What if a doctor instead said: "You're very seriously ill. I can operate on you, but in the end, it won't give you much more time. Everyone has the right to choose how they spend the time left to them."

If the physicians managing your care aren't willing to give you options in ways you understand, then you need to ask for someone else who can help you understand. The patient, as an educated consumer, must be prepared to seek out, initiate, and have those additional conversations. You must seek out a range of information and make the best decision based upon that information.

Question your physician. You don't have to have a medical background or know much about medicine to do that. I enjoy questions. That's why I'm the doctor with the chair. I shut off my phone, sit down, roll up to the patient so we can be face-to-face, and take questions. If she wants to talk for five minutes or four hours, I'm there for her. That way she's empowered to make the best decision for herself and her loved ones.

What specific questions can a patient or family ask to prevent treatments from steamrolling them? How can they prevent becoming confused and misled by medical terminology? What do they have a right to know?

Here are eight questions that every seriously ill patient and his or her family members should pose to their doctors:

1) In *your experience as a doctor*, will this treatment prolong my life? If so, for how long? At what physical and emotional cost?
Physicians like to speak in percentages based on research involving a cohort of patients. A trial may say 85% of patients showed positive results, while 15% were negative. But in

any individual situation, the percentage is fifty-fifty. As I've explained, patients tend to believe they will always be on the positive side of any percentage given to them. This requires that physicians be honest with patients and families **based on their knowledge and experience**. When the doctor tells a family, "I don't have a crystal ball," and then walks up to me and says, "Go tell them their father is dying," it is quite frustrating.

Ask doctors to be honest and specific:

- After the treatment, *in your experience*, how much time will I have left?
- If I cannot be cured, will I live longer with the treatment than if I didn't have it? How much longer? With the treatment, what is my quality of life expected to be?
- If I decline the treatment, how much time will I have left?

Don't accept a general answer or an evasion. Crystal balls are for mystics, not doctors. Ask the doctor to be specific: how many months or days do I have left to live? One study showed that oncologists told patients they had ninety days to live when, on average, the patients had about twenty-four days left.

2) Will this treatment improve my quality of life? In what ways?
Again, ask for and expect nothing less than specific and accurate information.

- *In your opinion*, what is the likelihood my husband/brother/wife/sister will be bedbound after the proposed surgery or treatment?

- Will they be able to feed themselves/toilet themselves/sit up in bed? Will they regain their cognitive functions?
- What is my chance of cure? What is the chance that this chemotherapy will make my cancer shrink? Stay stable? Grow?

Don't let your fear of the unknown prevent you from asking these hard questions.

The medical profession doesn't like confronting these kinds of questions. I've had patients who've just gotten out of the operating room after major surgery and their doctors don't want me to talk with them: "I've just done this amazing thing, putting them through hell to give them a fighting chance, and now you're going to go in there and tell them they're dying? No way."

I had a patient recently who epitomized the consequences of this aggressive, non-communicative approach. He was eighty-seven, had dementia, and lived at home. He was so debilitated that he couldn't be left alone. His family had hired a caregiver so he wouldn't burn down the house or walk into traffic.

One day, while walking outside with his caregiver, the patient fell and broke his neck. It was such a severe and unstable fracture that he risked death if he turned his head. He required very expensive surgery to fix his horrific injury; without it, he couldn't be able to get out of bed.

After the surgery, he had trouble swallowing without getting food into his lungs. His doctors weren't sure whether this was a temporary or permanent condition, so they spent three days conducting speech and swallow tests on him. He failed the tests miserably.

The doctors inserted a temporary feeding tube for a

couple of days. He was so demented that he kept pulling it out. A speech pathologist recommended that he get a permanent feeding tube because he couldn't eat or drink without it.

At this point, I got the phone call. The family didn't want the feeding tube because it wasn't the patient's wish. I talked with them, and they decided to take him home and make him comfortable for the remaining time he had left.

When the surgeon found out about this plan, he was not happy.

"I didn't operate on this patient just so he could go home and die," he told me. "I operated on him so he could go to rehab and return home."

But return home to what? I felt like asking. *So he could continue to live a demented life?*

The surgeon ordered another swallow test. The only point of it was to prove that the operation was "successful" and not in vain.

Had the family been empowered to ask questions, this torment might have been avoided. Ultimately the patient was discharged home with hospice, but that should have happened a lot earlier.

3) How much will this treatment cost? Is it covered by insurance? How much will I have to pay?

Make sure you know the cost of the procedure and whether your insurance will pay for it. Don't be shy about demanding this information. Why pay for a pointless medical treatment that will bankrupt your family, rob your children of their college funds, and fail to improve your quality of life? We ask about price in everything we do—mortgages, groceries, cable TV bills, hiring a handyman or contractor. Why do we not ask about price when it comes to our medical treatments? We can comparison shop for cat food, but we can't do the same for procedures that cost thousands of dollars?

4) What are the risks and side effects of this treatment?
With cancer patients, side effects can include nausea, vomiting, diarrhea, respiratory failure, heart failure, life-threatening anemia, and life-threatening infections. Many patients don't know or didn't hear the full ramifications of these side effects before agreeing to treatment.

Ask your doctor to be specific about side effects:

- What are the main side effects of the chemotherapy/ treatment/procedure? Will I feel better or worse?
- Do most patients suffer from them?
- How long do they last?
- How do you help treat the side effects?
- Also, ask about risks:
- What are the risks of the treatment? What are the likely things that will happen to me?
- Is there a chance I could pass away during the treatment? Is there a chance I could suffer bodily harm or loss of faculties from the treatment?
- What are the chances of me surviving the treatment? Of having a good quality of life after treatment?
- Can I speak to other patients with my condition? What have they experienced?

5) Would you still recommend this procedure if I die within thirty days and you're responsible for paying back the cost of the procedure to Medicare or other insurance companies as a result?

I'm completely serious—you should ask this question of your doctor(s). It can be asked in a light-hearted, humorous way if that makes it easier. The doctor's response will give you some sense of whether or not to go ahead with what he's recommending.

6) What are my other options if I don't choose this treatment? What about palliative care or hospice care at home?

Don't wait for your doctor to initiate a conversation about palliative or hospice care. If you're not proactive in starting that talk, you may be waiting a long time or suffer through unintended consequences. Ask direct questions:

- How do I explore hospice and palliative care options?
- Who can talk to me about them?
- When can I set up an appointment to talk about them?

Be sure to ask questions about the availability of hospice, even in the face of pressure to have more treatments.

One patient of mine was in the ICU on a ventilator. When he came off the machine, he and his wife agreed he was going to go home without a feeding tube, and his doctors weren't pleased: *He's going to be back here in two days, he's going to die in a week*, etc., etc.

His wife held her ground in the face of this pressure: "Absolutely not. He's not going to get a feeding tube, and he's not going back to another facility. I want him home."

He received hospice at home, and he lived an amazing life for another nine months. His wife attended to him 24/7 and he was able to eat and drink whatever he wanted. When he had problems with aspiration, hospice was there. When he developed a fever, he was started on an antibiotic.

He was bed-bound and couldn't clean himself after a bowel movement, but he and his wife were able to be with each other. They had a good time despite his circumstances. He was awake, he was alert, he was interactive, and they had great conversations. He achieved closure with his family. His quality of life improved, and as a result, he was able to live longer than expected. We worked with his family to help them with their grieving. He never went back to the hospital and died at home peacefully with his entire family by his side.

Hospice wasn't a "death sentence," as his doctors had predicted, simply because he didn't do what they wanted him to do.

7) Do I absolutely need all the medications I'm taking?

Patients with congestive heart failure have their lungs fill up with fluid, which causes shortness of breath and chest pain. The doctor will say, "Well, if you go home and you stop your diuretics, you're going to drown in your own fluids and not be able to breathe."

Hospice doctors don't talk that way. They use many medications in combination to help treat the pain and anxiety that accompany congestive heart failure. Patients don't drown in their fluids. They don't choke to death. They're never told that. Palliative care is presented to these patients in a different light. Because they understand that they're not going to go home and drown in their own secretions, they're more likely to accept such care sooner than later.

When patients start to decline, medication affects their ability to be awake all the time. It becomes a very fine line, because while I'm trying to treat their symptoms, I'm also trying to give them quality time with their families. I treat them in ways to relieve their symptoms without robbing them of the time they need with their loved ones.

You don't start people on medications that make them sleepy or unresponsive until they're in the active phase of dying. In the meantime, I want them to be able to participate in their family life. When the patient starts the final decline, we're not going to give her any more diuretics or antibiotics. I'll absolutely treat her symptoms, but in a way that gives her as much quality time as possible with family.

Here are questions to ask your doctor about medications:

- What are the side effects of my medications? For how long will I be on them?
- Will the medications make me drowsy or unresponsive?
- Do I need all the medications you have me on? Why?
- Are there alternatives to some or all of my medications? Are there other ways to relieve my pain?

8) Do you understand my wishes/my family's wishes for end-of-life treatment? Are you familiar with the advance directives I have in place?

If you don't have an advance directive or designated MPOA in place, then do so. Don't put it off any longer. Without such planning in place, medical decisions will be made for you when you can no longer make them for yourself. Don't wait until you're seriously ill.

Anyone can appoint a person to be his or her medical power of attorney by completing a form in the presence of two witnesses. This is critically important, and the form takes just a few minutes to fill out.

Talk to your doctor about end-of-life planning. A Danish study of 202 terminally ill patients found that those who planned for their deaths and discussed their preferences with their doctors lived longer than those who did not (*The Telegraph*, U.K., Dec. 10, 2019). Additional research has shown that patients who talk to their doctors about dying are more likely to reject high-risk treatments.

If you haven't done such planning already, it's never too late to begin. Ask these questions of your doctor:

- Do I need a will? Advance directives? How do I go about putting them in place? Who can I speak with?
- Should I appoint a medical power of attorney who can speak for me if I am unable? Should I appoint a durable power of attorney to handle my financial and legal affairs? How do I go about that?
- Will you help me talk with my children about my condition?
- Who is available to help me cope legally with my situation?

If you don't ask questions and make your wishes known, you're taking a huge risk. I had a patient who was clearly listed as "do not resuscitate/do not intubate," meaning no CPR and no ventilator. Unfortunately, when the patient arrived at the hospital, he was in extreme respiratory distress. The family was given an option: we can treat him or he will die. They were not given the option of comfort measures. I had to speak to the family the following day about the patient's wishes. We turned the ventilator off, and three hours later, the patient died peacefully in the intensive care unit.

In another case, I got called in to see a patient who had congestive heart failure and kidney disease. His kidneys were failing from the diuretics used to treat his heart failure, but when we stopped treating his heart failure, he had shortness of breath. It was a vicious cycle.

He had a very difficult heart rhythm and went into the hospital for a procedure to help with that. They ended up putting in a pacemaker/defibrillator, but it didn't improve his quality of life or functional status.

He told me, "I didn't want a defibrillator. Now I've got one that's keeping me alive. If my heart goes into a funky rhythm, it's going to shock me."

He got caught up in the system and was told he had to go back to rehab to improve his condition. He didn't want that. They ignored his wishes and scheduled the return to rehab. Finally someone called me.

"We're waiting for the psych people to evaluate him."

"What do you mean?"

"Well, after we told him he was going back to rehab, he slit his wrists."

The surgeon fixed his lacerations. After the surgeon left, the patient ripped open his wounds. The surgeon sewed him up a second time. Now the patient was under suicide watch.

I told his doctor, "He understands exactly what he wants, but he had to slit his wrists so someone would listen to him. This is a man who is thinking very clearly. Doesn't anyone understand that he has the mental capacity to not want CPR or to be put on a ventilator or to return to rehab?"

We were in this terrible place where a man was deemed incompetent when he truly understood what he wanted. But he had no advance directive. He had no medical power of attorney. If his heart went into a funky rhythm, he would get shocked and potentially end up in the ICU on a ventilator, exactly what he did not want. He would most likely die in the ICU.

He clearly qualified for and wanted hospice, but wasn't sent there. Instead, he was dispatched to the psych unit in the hospital. They spent a couple of days there working with him. They started him on an antidepressant and gave him some counseling. They concluded he was of sound mind and could make his own decisions. He said he wanted to go home with hospice, where he died the next day.

A terminal patient had to slit his wrists to get people to recognize and respect his wishes, when he could have been empowered in his choices from the beginning.

If your loved one never did any advance planning, has no directive or MPOA in place, and you never discussed your loved one's wishes for end-of-life care, you can ask yourself, family members, and friends the following questions to help decide what path to take, which can then be clearly communicated to your doctor.

- What was most important to mom? What would she say in this situation?
- Did she ever say anything about how she would want to be treated if she could no longer make decisions for herself?
- Did she ever talk about how friends or family were treated in her situation?
- What would she want in this situation, if she got sicker or the treatments didn't work?

When people start down the path of a terminal illness, they lose their independence. Dad may still be driving at ninety-two, but then he falls and breaks his hip. He has surgery and then has to live in a nursing home. He's not going home again. He gradually loses everything dear to him—his car, his home, his life with his family.

I tell patients and families this all the time: when you've lost your independence, when you're depending on people to feed you and help you with your bodily functions, picking how and where you're going to die can be the most empowering thing you'll ever do in life.

The most profound choice I can help a patient embrace is the ability to say, "I'm done with this. I'm taking control of my disease, and I'm going to die on my own terms."

CHAPTER NINE

Recommendations for Change

You don't go to medical school to learn how to help people die a comfortable death. You go to medical school to learn how to keep people alive at all costs.

Have I noticed changes in these attitudes? Are doctors becoming less inclined to urge aggressive treatments? Is there a shift occurring?

In my experience, some doctors I work with were trained before palliative care came to the forefront. Many of them are still reluctant to bring me in for the consult.

"They're not dying."

"Don't be a pessimist."

"They're not ready to give up."

Nevertheless, I have seen some incremental shifts in the hospitals and doctors I work with. Some hospitals are now looking at getting palliative care physicians involved sooner with severely ill patients and have created a tool for automatic palliative care referrals. If a patient has multiple comorbid conditions or multiple hospitalizations or has in-stage dementia or severe nutritional problems, he or she will be automatically referred.

In short, if you're a "high utilization" patient—you've been in the hospital multiple times, you've been in the ICU several times, you've been on a ventilator—it means you're a chronically ill patient who is at high risk. By automatically referring such patients to palliative care, you're not only treating them and their families in a more compassionate way, but saving the system thousands of dollars. By reducing high utilizers in the healthcare system, we can bring down costs and change the system from within. Study after study backs this up.

Medicare is implementing a reform designed to prevent chronically ill patients from returning to hospitals for repeat visits. If such a patient is treated in the hospital, discharged to their home or a facility, and then returns to the hospital within a certain period of time, it's called a "bounce back."

Medicare is now looking at penalizing systems for the bounce back. Medicare wants physicians and other providers to consider other options when treating terminal or chronically ill patients.

The oft-quoted definition of insanity is doing the same thing over and over again, always expecting and failing to achieve a different outcome. How, then, can we bring saner approaches to treating the terminally ill?

Here are my recommendations.

Mandatory courses in medical school on death and dying

When you look at the med school curriculum as it stands right now, there aren't many courses on death and dying, palliative care, or hospice. According to one study, medical students receive an average of seventeen hours in such courses during their four-year training. I was never offered a single such course during medical school. If you don't feel comfortable talking about mortality, you can't be an effective doctor.

But that's beginning to change. Hundreds of doctors at Massachusetts General Hospital in Boston are being trained to talk to seriously ill patients about their goals, values, and prognoses through the Serious Illness Conversation Guide, a script created by Drs. Atul Gawande and Susan Block at Ariadne Labs. The guide helps doctors conduct emotionally sensitive end-of-life conversations and has been used to train over 6,500 clinicians worldwide since 2012 (*The Washington Post*, Feb. 12, 2018).

In establishing a medical school course on death and dying, I think its timing is important. Med school starts with the sciences, the extreme granular detail of what you need to learn about medicine. That's not a time to be talking about death and dying because everybody's grinding through their studies. Most medical students wouldn't absorb the concepts of death and dying at this point in their training. The best time for a course would be when students are preparing to go out into their clinical rotations, spending a month with a cardiologist or an oncologist.

Such courses must be required. I read that one very prestigious medical school was excited about offering an elective in palliative care and end-of-life issues. But a single elective class isn't sufficient. I took an elective class in medical school on ethics. Think of the importance of that topic when it comes to medical practice. I was interested in the subject, so I chose to take the class. But why would the majority of med students pick an elective that would only add more work to their heavy schedules? That's why classes on death and dying should be mandatory, not optional.

Train doctors in effective communication skills

When you walk in the door with a white coat and a stethoscope around your neck, you have authority, power, and influence. That's true whether you're in your third year of medical school or have twenty-five years under your belt as a cardiologist. That's why I've said repeatedly in this book that doctors need to remember that we work for our patients, not the other way around.

To make that happen, it's crucial that we communicate effectively. A first-year resident may make a stray comment to a family about their loved one getting better, and the family will be grasping at that comment for the next month as I work with them.

And so, timing and choice of words are very important when doctors are preparing to have clinical contact. They need to understand larger goals that go beyond medically treating the patient.

Oncologists who practice and teach at the Johns Hopkins Kimmel Cancer Center have called on medical oncology training programs to invest substantially more time educating physicians in how to talk with terminal patients.

In a commentary published in the *Journal of Clinical Oncology* in April 2020, the physicians cited studies showing that cancer doctors deliver bad news to patients an average of thirty-five times a month while few have training in how to do it.

According to the researchers, oncology fellows engaged in lengthy post-doctoral training programs report getting more coaching on how to perform technical procedures than in how to conduct meetings with patients and families facing difficult choices.

As I've shown in this book, how doctors frame difficult

conversations has a profound influence on whether patients choose treatment or palliative care. I tell this to medical students and residents all the time—that they have an incredible responsibility to patients whose lives and deaths are in their hands. They need to use that power responsibly when they walk out of the classroom and into the hospital.

Physicians and other providers need to learn how to share information in clear and helpful ways. They need to learn how to listen, allow questions, allow silence, and how to sit with someone's sadness or anger. There's a technique called "motivational interviewing" that trains clinicians in ways that help ambivalent patients identify and overcome their reluctance in discussing end-of-life care.

Once they understand the huge responsibility they have, physicians and other providers should be taught how to present information in a way that doesn't bias the patient one way or the other. We have to be objective presenters of information and guide the patients objectively through their choices and options. We can't present procedures as either/or: either you have this procedure or you'll die.

When I worked as a police officer, I was a detective, and I got hours and hours of training on how to read a person. The spoken word is the smallest part of communication; most of what we say to one another is non-verbal. I learned how to read people's energy and body language to understand where they were coming from. I think medical students should receive similar training.

We also need to be more aware that some patients, no matter what words we use, have problems hearing us—literally.

In a 2016 survey of 510 hospice and palliative care providers across the U.S., 87% of them said they did not screen for hearing loss, even though 91% of them agreed that patients' hearing loss impedes conversation and negatively affects the quality of the care they receive. Only 61% said they felt confident that they could deal with patients with hearing problems (*Quartz*, Sept. 3, 2019).

This is another major deficit that needs to be addressed.

Improve ways doctors use language to discuss prognoses and other specific end-of-life issues

When a patient asks, "How much time do I have left?" almost every doctor will say, "I don't have a crystal ball, but I can tell you that we can continue to treat you and get you through this rough spot for a period of time."

When doctors say they don't have a crystal ball, I have to call bullshit on that. Doctors know when a patient is dying. It's difficult to predict when we continue to apply our technology, but pretty straightforward if we allow the natural course of the disease to progress.

I have to call bullshit when the patient doesn't have a chance to get through an illness and the doctors are saying she does. That's the part that's a little bit frustrating to me. Be honest with the patients to the best of your knowledge. That's all they want. I have heard countless times from patients and families: "You're the first doctor to actually say I'm dying. I knew I was, but nobody would say it!

Steps are being taken to address this problem. The Vermont Conversation Lab was created by Dr. Bob Gramling, a palliative care doctor, to study how physicians and other providers communicated with patients or family members around end-of-life issues (*Quartz*, Sept. 3, 2019). Gramling, whose father died from Alzheimer's, was struck by how sensitive he was to the words doctors used to discuss his dad's illness. The project recorded over 12,000 minutes of conversation involving 231 patients, which were then analyzed.

Bob's brother David, a professor of linguistics at the University of Arizona, aided in the study. More than a million words of conversation that took place over a two- to three-year period were studied for tone and speaking rhythm. It wasn't the words per se that were studied, but the emotion conveyed by the speakers and whether the speakers connected. A machine-learning algorithm was used to help automatically detect these moments of emotional connection.

Such studies can help doctors know what language to use, especially when a prognosis is uncertain. Going to extremes in one's choice of words is not helpful, i.e., "I don't have a crystal ball" vs. "You'll die without this treatment." Far better to say a procedure "won't be beneficial" rather than "it's futile."

There are so many specific scenarios where doctors can use better language. I've had many situations where a patient transitions from full resuscitation to DNR, and then a doctor comes in and says, "Oh, I saw that you transitioned to DNR. Do you understand that means we're not going to do this procedure or that procedure?" The patient then starts to question his or her decision, and a couple of days later, I get the call that the patient has changed back to full resuscitation and aggressive treatment. The sticker on the wrist that says "DNR" comes to be seen as a sign of failure, of giving up. A patient who originally comes in as DNR is not questioned as much as someone who changes to that status from full resuscitation, as if the patient doesn't have the cognitive or moral clarity to make that decision.

I've talked before about how the words we use can imply control and, with that, a false sense of responsibility. The words "do not resuscitate" can mean to many people, "don't treat me." Which implies that you have control over your impending death and that either you or your family member has to accept responsibility if you choose not to do something. Instead of being seen as an act of taking responsibility for how you die, DNR can seem to mean that it's your fault you're dying or that you don't have the will to fight.

For some patients, DNR means they're abandoning their families. It carries a tremendous amount of guilt. They feel horrible. "I've got a son that I'm never going to see graduate" or "I've got a son who's going to have kids, and I'll never get to see them." DNR comes to mean, "give up hope."

Again, our specific word choices can have a great impact. I was attending a seminar at a convention where the suggestion was made to change DNR to AND (Allow a Natural Death). If you're allowing a natural death to occur, you're not giving up. If you're allowing the course of events to naturally evolve, you're giving up the illusion that you have power over death. You're acknowledging what you can and can't control, which shifts the whole dynamic of death and dying.

I've read recently about another change in terminology: "withdraw care." When a patient's on a ventilator and there's no chance they're going to recover, the family can withdraw care and begin the transition to comfort measures. We're going to "compassionately extubate" the patient rather than simply take out the ventilator tube. We're not abandoning the patient; rather, with compassion, we're allowing an inevitable process to unfold, without guilt or stigma. Our choice of words plays a huge role in how we view and accept dying.

I had a patient in the ICU who wasn't able to make his decisions for himself. The room was filled with relatives when I arrived. We needed to discuss whether we would continue aggressive treatment or allow death to occur. We talked for a while, and then everyone left except for one family member, a woman who told me she was a communications teacher at a nearby medical school, teaching students how to talk about death and dying, and especially about how to communicate bad news. We had an illuminating conversation about our experiences.

Doctors need to be taught about what words to use and how to use them. It's crucial not to lead someone down the road of false hopes. Give them enough information in the right ways to make an informed choice, whatever it might be.

Teach doctors listening and self-reflective skills

Learning the skill of active listening helps doctors communicate in a way that balances their personal desire to save the world with taking into account what the patient wants. Active listening involves asking open-ended questions, such as "Tell me what happened" or "Help me understand," and repeating back to the speaker what was heard, to ensure mutual understanding.

We need to listen: that's what I tell the med school students and residents who rotate with me. When you're talking with a patient about a surgical procedure, are you listening to what the patient and family are saying to you? Are you noticing what is being said without words? Is everyone on the same page? What is not being said? What needs to be said?

In addition to listening skills, a doctor needs to be self-reflective: if I were talking to my terminally ill father, how would I present this information? Would I play God? Would I try to save the world? Would I convey false hopes to my dad? Or would I take a different approach? Would I be accepting of the belief that everyone dies and has the right to die a good death?

Ken Murray, Clinical Assistant Professor of Family Medicine at USC, authored a 2011 essay entitled "How Doctors Die: It's Not Like the Rest of Us, But It Should Be." Murray noted that most physicians forsake the end-of-life treatment they themselves offer their patients.

> What's unusual about them is not how much treatment they get compared to most Americans, but how little. For all the time they spend fending off the deaths of others, they tend to be fairly serene when faced with death themselves. They know exactly what is going to happen, they know the choices, and they generally have access to any sort of medical care they could want. But they go gently.

They're all too familiar with the expensive, grueling, and futile care that is routinely administered to terminal patients in the ICU.

> What [this treatment] buys is misery we would not inflict on a terrorist. I cannot count the number of times fellow physicians have told me, in words that vary only slightly, "Promise me if you find me like this that you'll kill me." They mean it. Some medical personnel wear medallions stamped "NO CODE" to tell physicians not to perform CPR on them. I have even seen it as a tattoo.

Teach patient responsibility

When I was in medical school, I attended a presentation where a doctor stated, "Genetics loads the gun and lifestyle pulls the trigger." That statement has stuck with me forever. Another way of saying it: man doesn't die of disease but commits suicide slowly through his lifestyle choices.

If you were financially responsible for your healthcare, would you eat better? Exercise more? Stop smoking? Reduce your alcohol intake? I always joke with friends when we're out to dinner and someone orders a hamburger or a sausage pizza: *that's what stents are for.*

People don't take care of themselves and end up in the hospital, but with the technology that exists today, they don't pay a high price for their bad behavior. They don't need their chests cracked open. The doctor sticks them in the leg, they get a stent inserted in their hearts intravenously, and they walk out the next day. Why should I change my eating habits and behavior when there's an easy fix and someone else is paying for it?

One insurance company offered an incentive: anyone who went for a physical and started treatment for an identified condition would receive a check for $500. Guess how many people took up the offer? Almost no one. But when the insurance company sent a $500 bill to anyone who hadn't had an annual physical, everyone showed up for one.

If a patient goes to a cardiologist, finds out he has heart disease, and gets a stent put in as an outpatient, that saves the system millions of dollars. If the patient doesn't find out he has a condition and ends up in the ER, that costs the system millions of dollars. Better yet—what if the patient exercised, didn't drink or smoke, and ate a healthy diet?

Other countries have a very different outlook than we do. They don't perform procedures past a certain point because it would bankrupt their health systems. There are many reasons for immense healthcare costs, but a large factor is that people aren't willing to change their lifestyles.

We need to find ways to make people more responsible for their healthcare.

Evaluate the costs of end-of-life treatments

I remember when Sarah Palin was talking about "death panels" in reference to Obamacare. There was a discussion about rationing end-of-life care, and she was saying that this would put your grandma to death. By distorting this subject through fear mongering, we lost the opportunity to have a much-needed frank conversation about how we treat death and dying in this country.

It wasn't a question of rationing healthcare, but evaluating whether it was futile to perform certain types of procedures on older and terminally ill patients who were in the last weeks of life. Palin's comments were similar to a commercial about alarm systems that depicts a violent home break-in to make the point. Sensationalism distorts our discussions.

Most people see the cost of healthcare as their main complaint, but what they're complaining about is their $100 co-pay, not the $50,000 surgery or the multi-million-dollar ICU or the hundreds of thousands of dollars' worth of equipment they're plugged into. That's all being paid for by insurance. We complain about our personal costs but not the societal costs.

Litigation attorneys want their fee up front. Physicians don't ask for that. When someone goes into a hospital, no one asks, "How are you going to pay this bill?" Physicians don't do things for money, but in other countries they don't do certain procedures near the end of life. Can we bring financial reforms to our system or is it always going to be out of control? Should we bring rationing to the system? Is there an ethical issue involved in withholding certain treatments?

I'm not in favor of rationing healthcare because it sounds like we're depriving someone of a treatment they need. Instead, I think we need to look at ways we can be more reasonable with healthcare dollars. When you have your house painted, you get bids from three people. We need to bring the same competition to healthcare.

We know that when people have to do something more than once a day, they're more non-compliant. I can give you a pill that you're supposed to take three times a day, with each pill costing five cents. Or you can take a pill once a day that costs $5. Or one drug might have a 20% better chance of a positive outcome than another drug, but it costs $2,000 per month. What is the best option in that situation, taking into account both cost and effectiveness?

We have patients coming into hospice who take twenty or thirty pills daily—Pills that treat conditions and pills that treat the side effects of other pills. The list goes on and on. When they come into hospice, we trim those down significantly.

When a patient is terminal, it doesn't matter whether he or she is taking medications that cost $5,000 a month or $5 a month. When it's time, they're going to die. In my experience, I rarely see a patient take a sudden turn for the worse because they were transitioned to a less costly medication or because a medication was discontinued altogether.

On top of prices for medication, there's the cost of your dysfunctional and bloated healthcare system that is wedded to private insurance companies.

Every year, Americans collectively pay about $500 billion in administrative costs for healthcare—that is, for things like billing and insurance overhead, not for actual medical care.

These costs are significantly higher than in most other wealthy countries. One study on healthcare data from 1999 showed that each American paid about $1,059 per year just in overhead costs for healthcare; in Canada, the per capita cost was $307. Those figures are likely much higher today (Farhad Manjoo, *The New York Times*, Dec. 4, 2019).

Bring quality of life into the discussion

We need to make a shift from a "fix it at all costs" mentality to a medical system based on well-being.

I don't believe in rationing healthcare or drawing a line for treatments at a certain age. Instead, I would look at the totality of the situation. Are people living better and longer lives after receiving dialysis at an advanced age? Some people in their eighties and early nineties do well on dialysis for a period of time before they don't do well.

So I wouldn't say we should withhold dialysis because you're eighty-five years old. Instead, we should look at each case on an individual basis. What is the person's current functional status? Will dialysis improve that status? Will they be able to resume a quality life after treatment, or will their existence be limited to wearying trips to a dialysis center? Is the patient being told that he or she has the option to stop treatment? Or are they being misled?

Empower patients to ask questions and make knowledgeable choices

This book is about empowering people. The medical establishment has its own logic and momentum, but it's the patient who has the power to say no (or the power to be educated to say no). If more patients are educated and physicians are more sensitive to this issue, then patients will have the freedom of more options.

We can reform the medical establishment up to a point, but it doesn't seem like we're going to go to a Canadian system or something like a single-payer system anytime soon. Instead, the patient has to be put in the driver's seat. Realistic reform is really about making sure the patient holds the power.

And that means being aware of how doctors view their jobs and how they communicate. It means being aware that you have the right to palliative and hospice care, so that someone like me can be brought into the picture sooner than later.

Put palliative care and hospice care at the forefront

According to a recent survey by the Center to Advance Palliative Care (CAPC), nearly 80% of consumers who received information about palliative care said they would choose it for themselves or their loved ones. The figure jumps to 87% for survey respondents over age sixty-five. Yet, about 71% of Americans have little to no understanding of what palliative care is (*Journal of Palliative Medicine*). And close to 60% of patients who would benefit from palliative care never receive it (*New England Journal of Medicine*).

We are also facing a shortage of trained hospice and palliative care physicians. An estimated 10,000 people in the U.S. become Medicare-eligible each day, a trend that many expect to continue until 2029, according to the Medicare Payment Advisory Commission (MedPac). And yet we face a shortage in hospice and palliative care specialists for adults sixty-five and older, according to an April 2018 study by the National Center for Biotechnology Information. The research estimated that by 2040, we'll need 10,640 to 24,000 such specialists, when actual supply is expected to range between 8,100 and 19,000. The study also showed that hospice and palliative care providers are facing shortages in chaplains, nurses, and social workers.

We need to bring the practice of palliative care into all specialties. It can be practiced by all doctors, not just those who specialize in it.

I was recently recruited by a facility that specializes in cancer care. They were working on getting their Medicare certification and needed a palliative care doctor. Several different people in their system interviewed me, and one of them was an oncologist. As I sat across from him, he spun his computer screen around so I could see it.

"Every one of the patients on this list has Stage 4 cancer," he said. "They're terminal patients and they're not going to be cured. We're just treating them right now."

He paused to make sure his next point got across.

"Number one, I'll tell you when it's time for you to have your talk. Number two, I'll tell you what to say, what topics you can discuss, and what topics you can't discuss. And then I'll make the final decision about whether the patient continues to be treated or not."

I couldn't believe what I'd heard.

I bit my tongue, looked past his cavalier comments, thanked him for the opportunity, and declined the offer.

Remove financial rewards for pointless treatments

If a physician administers $18,000 worth of medication and the patient dies a month later, shouldn't that doctor be liable for paying back that $18,000 to Medicare? If physicians were liable in that way, might they think twice about administering some treatments? Would they be confident about advocating for an aggressive approach?

Medicare also tells me that if I keep someone in hospice for more than six months, I'm going to be penalized and pay them back for the services I provided. Why should a hospice physician be penalized for providing end-of-life care, but a provider not be liable for administering treatment to a patient who has no chance of survival?

If the provider faced the same liability that I face, he might have a different approach with his patient: "You know what? I'm not going to stick a tube into your chest today to drain fluid. I'm not accomplishing anything. I think it's time to talk with you and your family about better options at this point in time."

Physician-assisted suicide is a sign of failure

For most people, physician-assisted suicide is linked with empowerment. When someone has a terminal illness and has lost all independence, when their quality of life has declined to the point where they no longer want to live, such a person may want the power to choose to end his or her life.

In order to qualify for physician-assisted suicide in states where it's legal, you need to pass psychiatric and medical evaluations. It has to be clear that you're aware of the decision that you're making and that other treatment options are available.

The bottom line is about empowering someone to have ultimate control, and yet the reality is that very few people opt for physician-assisted suicide. In fact, most people who qualify for the program never go forward with it.

I see physician-assisted suicide as a failure of the system. We've failed to educate the person about dying. We've failed to provide them with other options. That's what hospice is about. It's working with people—recognizing their fears, addressing those fears, and empowering them to face their choices with as little fear and pain as possible.

The mere act of choosing to die in a hospital or at home

gives someone power. It's a decision that no one else can make for you. If you pick the time of your mortality, if you allow the disease to run its course while you're also addressing your physical and psychosocial needs, that's true empowerment. Which is why I view physician-assisted suicide and suicide in general as failures. It's the only option a person has when he's hopeless, helpless, and not empowered.

When you look at suicide statistics, there are far more unsuccessful attempts than successes. That's because most attempts at suicide are cries for help. The person didn't want to die; he or she wanted attention that was lacking. Physician-assisted suicide is a sign that we're not giving people the attention, compassion, and empowerment they need. In a medical system that had more of those qualities, such an option would be very rare or unnecessary.

Remove taboos about discussing death

There has to be a general acknowledgment among doctors that we're all dying from the day we're born. If we deny that unalterable fact, we lose the ability to bring true compassion and caring into our profession. We can slow the dying process, but we can't defeat death.

Fear of death can cause us to make unwise and counterproductive choices in how we face illness and dying. Instead of being afraid of death, we should become comfortable with it. We should bring awareness and acceptance of it into our daily lives. We'd have much more gratitude for our lives and the people around us. We'd be preparing for our deaths in a much healthier and kinder way.

There are many efforts underway to bring dying and death into the public discourse and help people talk about it.

The Conversation Project (https://theconversationproject.org) helps people talk about their wishes for end-of-life care. Death Cafes have sprouted up around the country (https://deathcafe.com), where people gather to discuss death in an effort to make the most of their finite lives. Death over Dinner (https://deathoverdinner.org) is an international movement: thousands of people in over twenty countries have gathered to dine and discuss their views about "dying a good death." At Memorial Sloan Kettering Hospital in New York City, doctors, nurses, patients, and caregivers meet on a regular basis for Death over Dinner conversations centered on end-of-life issues.

Epilogue

I'll end this book with one last story, about a ninety-year-old man with cardiac problems. Harvey came into the hospital, they put in stents, and they sent him home. He was back in four days. They put in a pacemaker. He went home and came back again in a week. They put him on medication and kept him in the ICU. He went home and a few days later was once again back in the hospital.

After he'd gone through that cycle about five times, I got the phone call. When I met with him, he said, "You know, they're telling me to do all these things. The best I can do is get home for three or four days, and then I'm right here back in the hospital. This is no life. So what can you do for me?"

"We can get you out of here and get you home," I said, "where we can keep you comfortable. Now, you may die in a week or two. Or it might be even longer. But during that time, my job will be to make sure that you don't have difficulty breathing, don't have chest pain, and don't have anxiety. You won't have those things that keep driving you back to the hospital."

Harvey told me, "That's exactly what I want to do."

He went home and chose to end all medications except for those that made him comfortable. About two weeks later, he passed away. When his daughter called me to give me the news, I asked her how it went.

"We were at home, and he was sitting in his chair watching TV," she told me. "We were having an amazing conversation and he asked if he could have a cup of coffee. I went into the kitchen, got the coffee, and brought it back out to him. While I was gone, he had passed away in his chair. And so peacefully. He had no difficulty breathing. He had none of the pain that he had been so afraid of."

The oncologist or the nephrologist or the cardiologist is not my enemy. He may have given my hospice patient six or seven more years of life, an immeasurable, priceless gift. In this way, the family will always know that the doctor never gave up. The doctor will have the everlasting respect of the family.

But neither is death the enemy. The oncologist may have had many successes in treating my hospice patient, but he didn't fail when there was nothing more he could do. At some point, inevitably, for all of us, disease overtakes any treatment that exists. The patient's death is as emotionally damaging to the physician as it is to the family. I know this from hard-won personal and professional experience. You feel as if you've failed. You feel you could have done more. You wish you had done things differently. The emotional impact on doctors is huge and can lead to burnout, but a natural death is not a failure. What we *do* fail at is helping people die a good death.

We need time to prepare for the emotional consequences of death. If a physician is hesitant to initiate or even accept the planning needed for that preparation, we're cheating the people in our care. If we're sensitive to the realities of dying and can talk honestly to patients about those realities, we're not going to take their precious time away from them. We're not going to put them in the intensive care unit in their final weeks.

Hospice uses well that precious time. It's not a place where people go to die but rather a place where people learn to die, to find peace with their mortality. And we help the family find that peace as well.

We can't do that in a day. We can't do that in a week. We can't do that in three months. No one can prepare to face their mortality with dignity and courage in such a short length of time.

My role as a hospice doctor is not to stop someone's treatment. Rather, I'm there to start a new conversation. The doctor has done all he can—he's given someone another seven years of life. I can now provide an experience that's just as positive. I can relieve the doctor from any sense of failure and guilt, just as I can relieve the family from that same burden.

Yet, I'm still called "Dr. Death" by some of my colleagues. I'm still greeted with "here comes the Grim Reaper" when I walk into the doctor's lounge. It's said tongue in cheek, as a form of jest, but it always disturbs me deep in my core. Most doctors don't wake up every day knowing that they will be associated with death during their daily rounds; rather, they're seen as the good guys, the knights in shining white coats, the heroes who preserve life against all odds.

I will always find that shocking. My unwanted nickname epitomizes all of the problems we create in treating the terminally ill. I hope I've explained why and how that treatment must change. Perhaps someday, doctors, patients, and families will no longer view death and dying as the enemy. Maybe we'll find more compassionate ways to deal with our feelings about our common mortality and how we face death when it comes.

The positive news is that we're slowly moving in that direction. Just before I finished this book, Doctor X, who I referred to in the introduction, stopped me in the hallway of the hospital one morning.

"Ken, can you go see one of my patients and have a talk with him? He's ready for you." He paused a moment, then added: "By the way, you're not Doctor Death—to me, you're Doctor Comfort."

It wasn't the right moment to discuss the ways the medical system needs to change or how we could mutually support one another in the work we do. Perhaps someday the two of us will have that conversation in depth. Instead, I simply thanked him and headed off down the hallway to see our patient.

Acknowledgments

I want to express deep gratitude to Megan, my fiancé. Without your push to "stop talking about it and DO it," this book would never have been written. Your constant love and encouragement kept me motivated through countless late nights and early mornings. When I doubted or questioned myself, you were always there to offer positive support. By reviewing my manuscript over and over again, you provided honest and sometimes painful feedback that made this book the best it could be. I love you.

Many thanks also to Al Desetta (www.aldesetta.com), whose writing and editing skills were instrumental in this project.

Resources for Readers

Healthcare Planning

https://www.americanbar.org/groups/law_aging/resources/health_care_decision_making/

Raising Awareness about Death

The Conversation Project (https://theconversationproject.org) helps people talk about their wishes for end-of-life care.

Death Cafes (https://deathcafe.com/) help people gather to discuss death in an effort to make the most of their finite lives.

Death over Dinner (https://deathoverdinner.org) enables groups to discuss their views about "dying a good death."

About the Author

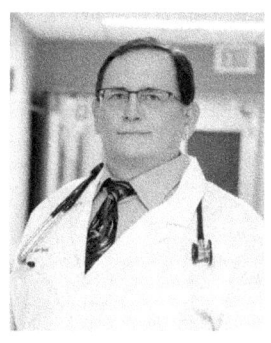

Dr. Ken Pettit was born in Baldwin Park, Cal. and raised in Gilbert, Az. First exposed to medicine as a hospital orderly at age 18, he worked as an EMT before becoming a police officer and later a detective. After leaving law enforcement, Pettit obtained intermediate EMT and paramedic certifications, working in emergency rooms as an ER technician.

He earned an associate degree in nursing at Excelsior College and worked as an RN for several years, before going on to medical school at Western University of Health Sciences, College of Osteopathic Medicine of the Pacific, in Pomona, Cal. He completed his residency at Midwestern University in Glendale, Az. Dr. Pettit is Board Certified by the American Osteopathic Board of Family Physicians, with a Subspeciality Board Certification in Hospice and Palliative Medicine. He is also a Certified Hospice Medical Director by the American Academy of Hospice and Palliative Medicine.

For 15 years Dr. Pettit worked in family practice, urgent care, and wound care before transitioning fulltime to hospice and palliative care. He has received a number of awards for his work. For recreation he enjoys riding Harleys, flying helicopters, and travel.

Index

advance directives, 44–45,
    60–68, 117–118
advance planning. *see* advance
    directives
aggressive treatment, 3, 33,
    42–43, 60, 87,
    129–130
AI (artificial intelligence),
    101–102
Annals of Internal Medicine, 47
anticipatory grief, 14
aphasia, expressive, 106
Arizona state
    law, 26, 64
    providing caregiving for
        indigent person, 25
    surrogate decision-making
        in, 63–64
arrhythmia, 96
aspiration, 28, 106, 107, 118
    handling patients with,
        28–30
automatic palliative care
    referrals, tool for,
    123–124

"bounce back", 124

Cabbage Patch, 59
caregivers, 25, 90, 105–106, 112,
    141
chaplain, 2, 13, 99
chemotherapy, 4, 11, 24, 50, 74,
    75, 81, 114
    cost of, 93, 94, 95, 100
chronically ill patients. *see*
    "super-utilizers"
comfort care. *see* palliative
    care
comfort measures, 2, 43, 118,
    130
comfort treatment, 90, 108
communication, non-verbal, 48,
    61, 90, 127
conservative management,
    109
Conversation Project, 141
COPD (chronic obstructive
    pulmonary disease),
    15, 96
cost
    evaluation of end-of-life
        treatments, 134–135
    for healthcare in U.S.,
        93–94

courses in medical school
    on death and dying, 124–125
Covid-19 pandemic, 4
CPR, 17, 22, 51, 58, 65, 71, 80
Curtis, Randall, 44

death, 3, 6
    courses in medical school, 124–125
    emotional consequences of, 144
    fear of, 140
    natural, 4, 130
    nonverbal communication about, 61
    panels, 134
    removing taboos about discussing, 140–141
    slipshod preparation for, 33
    talk, 77–91
Death Cafes, 141
Death over Dinner, 141
deception, case examples for, 21–35
defibrillator, implantable, 96–98, 100, 119
denial, case examples for, 21–35
divine intervention, power of, 87
doctors
    improving ways to use language to discuss prognoses, 128–131
    palliative care, 47
    patient's or family member's questions to, 110–118
    responsibilities, 6, 41, 43, 74, 83, 94, 105–107
    teaching to listening and self-reflective skills, 131–132
    training in effective communication skills, 126–128
dysfunction
    case examples for, 21–35
    degree of, 63

empowerment of patients, 34, 78, 107
    to ask questions and make knowledgeable choices, 136–137
end-of-life, 3. *see also* experiences of doctors with end-of-life patients
    care, 28, 120, 138–139
    cost evaluation of treatments, 134–135
    decisions, 30, 61–64
    documents, 60
    existential crisis, 49
    issues, 78, 128–131
    patient's activities near, 67
expensive life-prolonging treatment. *see also* Medicare—hospice benefits
    angioplasty, 93–94
    chemotherapy, 93
    implantable defibrillator, 96–98

Index

experiences of doctors with end-of-life patients
    dealing with family members, 15–20
    dealing with patients without knowing hospice care, 9–15
    handling patients with aspiration, 28–30
    MPOA issue of family members, 24–28
extended prognosis, 100

family dysfunction, 21–24, 30–33
financial liability, 95, 100
financial rewards removal for pointless treatments, 138–139

"getting better", patients believing, 37–40, 45–55, 83–84
Gramling, Dr. Bob, 128
group home, 43, 100

hope, 39, 49, 94–95, 102, 131
hospice care, 3–4, 6, 13, 43, 115–116, 144
    complaint about, 102
    managing medications in, 82
    patient's questions about, 110–111
    putting at forefront, 137–138
hospice companies, 40, 102

hospice patients, 43, 82
hypothermia protocol, 17

IDT (interdisciplinary team) meeting, 40
Impella device, 73
insanity, 124
Isaac, Margaret, 44

Journal of Palliative Medicine study, 3

Kaiser Family Foundation poll report, 3
Knoll, Herb, 14

Left Ventricular Assist Device (LVAD), 73
life-prolonging system, 3. *see also* expensive life-prolonging treatment

Markam, Dr. Anil, 43–44
medical establishment, 3, 102–103, 136
medical power of attorney (MPOA), 6, 24–28, 58, 60–61, 63–64
medical technology, 69–76
Medicare, 40, 93, 94, 124, 138
    conclusions about hospice, 102
    guidelines, 101
    hospice benefits, 99–100
medications, 16, 69, 71, 82, 91, 98
    questions to ask doctor about, 117

National Center for Biotechnology Information (NCBI), 45
research, 42
National Hospice and Palliative Care Organization (NHPCO), 3–4, 102
New England Journal of Medicine, 3
nurses, 10, 13, 27, 48–49, 91, 99

opioid crisis, 44

palliative care, 3–4, 42–43, 115–116
   consultation, 44
   doctors/physicians, 30, 47, 71
   integration of, 44
   patient's questions about, 110–111
   providers, 127
   putting at forefront, 137–138
patient responsibility, teaching, 132–133
patient's or family member's questions
   about cost of treatment, 113–114
   about doctor's experience, 110–111
   about need of medications, 116–117
   about palliative care or hospice care, 115–116
   about recommendation of treatment, 114–115
   about risks and side effects of treatment, 114
   about treatment quality, 111–113
   about wishes for end-of-life treatment, 117–118
physician-assisted suicide, 139–140
physicians. *see* doctors
physician's assistant (P.A.), 10
pre-grief. *see* anticipatory grief
"pulling the plug" issue of "killing mom", 65, 67

quality of life, 44, 70–71, 95–96, 111–113, 136

recommendations for change
   bringing quality of life into discussion, 136
   empowering patients to ask questions and make knowledgeable choices, 136–137
   evaluating costs of end-of-life treatments, 134–135
   improving ways to doctors use language to discuss prognoses, 128–131
   mandatory courses in medical school on death and dying, 124–125

physician-assisted suicide, 139–140
putting palliative care and hospice care at forefront, 137–138
removing financial rewards for pointless treatments, 138–139
removing taboos about discussing death, 140–141
teaching doctors to listening and self-reflective skills, 131–132
teaching patient responsibility, 132–133
training for doctors in effective communication skills, 126–128
religious belief of patients and families, 86–88
resuscitation, 22, 25, 50, 64–65, 80, 129

severely ill patients. *see* terminal patients
social worker, 2, 13, 66, 99, 137
suffering, 2, 3, 5, 19, 33, 87, 96, 97, 106, 114
"super-utilizers", 94
SUPPORT Act (2018), 98
supportive care. *see* palliative care
surrogate decision-making, 63–64

taboos removal about discussing death, 140–141
terminal diagnosis, 43
terminally ill patient. *see* terminal patients
terminal patients, 2, 4, 13, 14, 34, 40, 61, 93, 107, 118, 123, 126, 132, 134, 138
tracheostomy, 53, 59, 62, 80, 89

The Widower's Journey (Knoll), 14

www.ingramcontent.com/pod-product-compliance
Lightning Source LLC
LaVergne TN
LVHW011708060526
838200LV00051B/2812